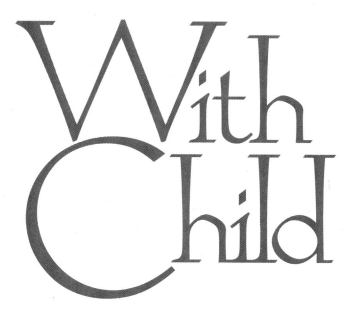

With Child

Created by
Jamie Eloise Bolane, B.F.A.

Illustrated by
Bernie Kida, C.M.I.
Kent Boughton, M.S., C.M.I.
Karen Martin, M.F.A.

Designed by
Stephen Ott

a publication of

**CHILDBIRTH
GRAPHICS®**

a division of WRS Group, Ltd.
Waco, TX 76702-1207

43317-6009-0999

©1995, 1999 Childbirth Graphics®, a division of WRS Group, Ltd.

First published in the United States of America in 1995 by Childbirth Graphics®,
a division of WRS Group, Ltd., P.O. Box 21207, Waco, Texas 76702-1207
800-299-3366 ext. 287

10 9 8 7 6 5 4 3 2

Bolane, Jamie Eloise.
    With child / created by Jamie Eloise Bolane; illustrated by
Bernie Kida, Kent Boughton, Karen Martin; designed by Stephen Ott.
        p.   cm.
    Includes bibliographical references.
    ISBN 1-56796-135-5
    1. Pregnancy--Popular works. 2. Childbirth--Popular works.
    I. Title.
RG525.B64427   1995
618.2--dc20   95-41110
                                                                                  CIP

ISBN 1-56796-135-5

to Rusty
for his love and endurance

and to our children
Holly, Christopher, Peter, and Jesse

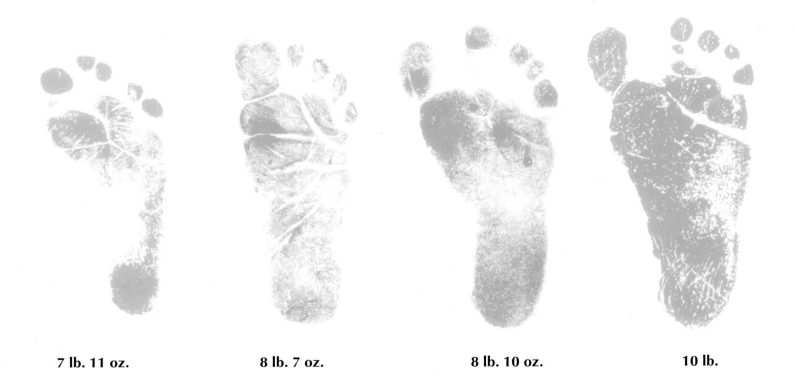

7 lb. 11 oz.   **8 lb. 7 oz.**   **8 lb. 10 oz.**   **10 lb.**

(all full-term babies)

Acknowledgments

This book stands on the shoulders of many determined people. My first teachers were expectant parents themselves when I began working in birth education in 1968. My efforts have been continually informed by three remarkable women: Eunice (Kitty) Ernst, CNM, of the National Association of Childbearing Centers, Ruth Watson Lubic, CNM, EdD, of the Maternity Center Association in New York, and Harriette Hartigan, midwife, writer, photographer, and friend. Together they have permanently altered my comprehension of the experience of childbearing as one that transforms and empowers a woman's life. They taught me reverence for nature's incredible design that enables a woman's body to nurture and give birth to a new human being. They taught me the value of sheltering and supporting new families so they can adjust to the demanding roles of parenting. And they taught me that midwives are among the keepers of the light. My share of the profits of this book will be divided equally among these three women in appreciation of their work. May they continue to inform and inspire others.

My ability to conceive of this publication began with the formation of Childbirth Graphics in 1980. In its first years it was a "made with love" company that grew solely through the dedication of those who worked with me from their homes: Susan Lange, Carolyn Kerhaert, Nancy Johnson, Ginny Miers, and Nancy Jacobsen. Their devotion to what we were trying to accomplish made all that has followed possible. With Child incorporates the essence of many products from those years, created with love by the many staff members who followed. Everything we achieved was based on what the birth educators in this country told us that they needed.

In the early 1990s I reached a point where the principle elements of this and other publications were in my head, yet they were never going to come together if I could not free myself from the relentless demands of running a business. I was given the expertise and resources of Tucker Capital Corp. in finding a new owner for Childbirth Graphics. Kemp Battle spent endless hours caring enough to fully comprehend our unique business so that he could find a company that would fit our complex operation of product development, print production, model manufacturing, and catalog marketing and distribution. Over a long year we found the situation that would give me the freedom to return to creative thinking. His tireless efforts were backed by Craig Battle, David Baxendale, and Stephanie Beddows.

In 1992 Childbirth Graphics moved to Texas and became part of the WRS Group of health related companies. I am grateful for the full support that Wayman Spence, MD, Jary Ganske, and Leonard Hooks have given my ideas for educational materials. Barbara Silcox, Linda Filgo, and Stephen Ott demonstrated remarkable patience while I worked and reworked the evolution of With Child. The artists Bernie Kida, Karen Martin, and Kent Boughton listened and responded to what I wanted to convey in each illustration and then added their many talents to create the lasting images in this book. Finally, a special thank you to the editorial staff Jules Robinson, Steve Toon, and Shane Petty for their excellent work, and to Brenda Roberts and Pam Schreiber for their research on the resources section.

My family simply endured. My husband Rusty stood behind the travel, the conferences, the meetings, and the endlessly unpredictable schedules and underestimated hours of work. Our children Holly, Christopher, Peter, and Jesse grew up being exposed to more visual information on birth than most people receive in a lifetime. Their love has sustained me.

Table of contents

Genetics and reproduction

1 Month

2 Months

3-4 Months

5-6 Months

Newborn— the first days

Parenting and breastfeeding

Postpartum

Reading and video resources for child-bearing

Bibliography

Resource organizations

Preconception planning

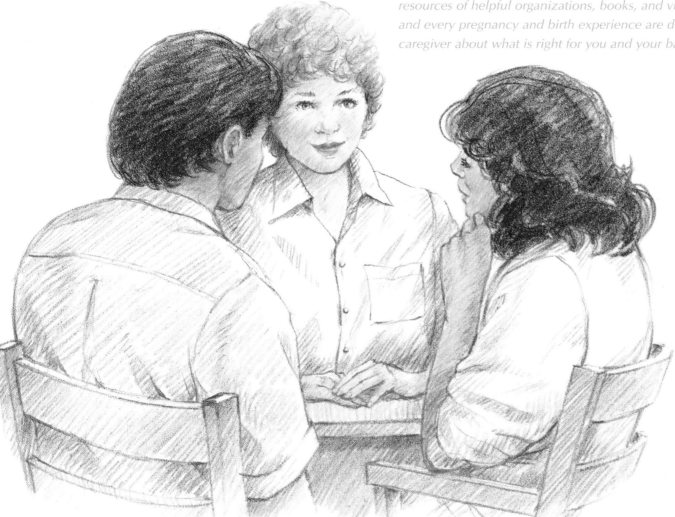

This book offers you information and suggestions for making healthy choices before you are pregnant, while you are pregnant, and in the first weeks after you give birth. Additional resources of helpful organizations, books, and videos are provided as well. Every woman and every pregnancy and birth experience are different. Always consult your personal caregiver about what is right for you and your baby.

Childbearing today

Conceiving a child, being pregnant, giving birth, and welcoming a new life are all normal, healthy, human events. Yet, few moments in our lives have such capacity to change us forever. While the actual process of giving birth remains the same, our understanding of genetics, fertility, and fetal development is expanding almost daily. Scientists and medical professionals are beginning to appreciate just how critical the first weeks of pregnancy are for the developing embryo. Your state of health and your partner's state of health *before* you conceive can have permanent effects on your pregnancy and your developing baby. You are making lifestyle and health choices every day. If you are trying to conceive a child, they can be some of the most important choices you make.

3

Preconception planning: lifestyle changes before you are pregnant

You and your partner have established a lifestyle that is comfortable. What many potential parents do not realize is that activities that may be acceptable for their life before pregnancy may have the potential to cause permanent harm to a developing fetus. All of a baby's major organs, such as its brain, heart, and lungs, will form in the first 12 weeks of pregnancy. They are at the greatest risk for damage during a period of time when many women may not be aware that they are pregnant. Getting healthy and staying healthy while you are trying to become pregnant and throughout your pregnancy can help prevent birth defects.

Preconception medicine

A new medical specialty, known as preconception medicine, offers prepregnancy planning. Specially trained physicians can evaluate your health and your partner's health and make recommendations to give you the best chance to conceive and carry a healthy child. They can help you decide if you need to have genetic testing and counseling before you conceive. Couples should think about where they work, what they eat, and what changes they might make in their lives *before* they try to become pregnant. Changing your lifestyle before you conceive is an important decision. What can you and your partner do to help prepare for a healthy pregnancy and birth?

Physical readiness

Before trying to conceive, have a physical exam to discuss your general health and any medical history of sexually transmitted diseases, stillbirth, miscarriage, and chronic health conditions such as diabetes or high blood pressure. Have routine screening tests for possible infections—particularly sexually transmitted diseases.

Psychological readiness

A baby will change your lifestyle as well as your relationships with your partner, your friends, and your parents. Talk with your partner about what each of you expect. What makes you comfortable? What do you fear the most? What kind of parents do you want to be for your child? How will you handle the costs? Will you be able to stay at home with your baby? Where can you find competent and loving day care?

Weight

Studies show that being significantly overweight or underweight may complicate your pregnancy. Ask your healthcare provider about your ideal weight and how to achieve it.

Nutrition

Eating for two doesn't mean eating twice as much—it means eating twice as well. If you are not in the habit of eating well, you should get into the habit now, before you get pregnant. Start by replacing junk food and empty calories with healthy food choices. Also drink plenty of water.

Prenatal vitamins

Prenatal vitamins contain special nutrients such as folic acid that are important during pregnancy in preventing some forms of birth defects. It is recommended that you begin taking prenatal vitamins before you conceive. Ask your healthcare provider about getting a prescription.

Education

There is so much to understand about your pregnancy and your growing baby. Prenatal classes will help you identify the choices you are making. Some communities offer prepregnancy planning education classes through private instructors, birth centers, or hospitals.

Exercise

Exercising before and during pregnancy offers many benefits to both mother and baby. If you are not normally active, consult with your healthcare provider before beginning an exercise program.

X-rays

Even small particles of radiation can harm a developing fetus. If either partner needs to have an X-ray for any reason, always tell the X-ray technician that you are trying to conceive a baby or that you are pregnant. If you are pregnant and an X-ray is unavoidable—even dental X-rays—insist on having your abdomen covered with a protective shield during the procedure.

On-the-job radiation exposure

If you work in any environment which exposes you to X-rays or radioactive material, notify your healthcare provider. You may need to change job assignments while you are trying to conceive and while you are pregnant.

Lead dust exposure

Many older homes and apartment buildings still have lead based paints in them. As the paint ages, it creates a dust that you can easily pick up on your hands. Interior and exterior paint can have lead in it. Avoid contact with lead dust or lead based paints and wash your hands frequently. When your baby is born, you will need to be extra careful to wipe lead paint surfaces clean. Lead dust can cause sickness and even brain damage in growing children.

Immunizations

If you've never had German measles, you should get a vaccination at least three months before you attempt to get pregnant. Measles during pregnancy can result in birth defects and miscarriage. Your healthcare provider may recommend other immunizations.

Recreational drugs

Social drugs can damage sperm or eggs and have devastating effects on a growing fetus. If either you or your partner uses drugs, stop now or get into a program to help you stop.

Sexually transmitted diseases

If you have or suspect you might have a sexually transmitted disease (STD), be sure that you tell your healthcare provider and get treatment. Some STDs can make it difficult for you to conceive. Other STDs may cause severe damage to your baby while in the womb or during birth. Even if you have an STD that can't be cured, there are treatments that can help to prevent your baby from being infected or harmed.

Smoking and secondhand smoke

Women who smoke have a harder time getting pregnant than nonsmokers; men who smoke can have low testosterone levels and a low sperm count. Babies born to smoking mothers have a lower average birthweight, weaker lungs, and a higher risk of problems than those born to non-smokers. If you smoke, get help to quit now. Avoid exposure to secondhand smoke before and during pregnancy.

Smokeless tobacco

Nicotine and other chemicals in chewing tobacco or snuff can be just as harmful to a developing fetus as cigarettes.

Alcohol

Alcohol use can reduce a couple's ability to conceive a baby. During pregnancy, there is no safe level of alcohol consumption. A pregnant woman's alcohol use can cause fetal alcohol syndrome (FAS), a condition characterized by growth retardation, facial abnormalities, and central nervous system dysfunction.

Caffeine

The issue of caffeine intake during pregnancy continues to be a controversial one. Although some studies have shown that too much caffeine may affect fertility and may not be safe for a fetus, moderate caffeine intake during pregnancy is generally considered safe. It is important to remember, however, that products containing caffeine (coffee, tea, colas, and chocolate) are not the most nutritious food and drink choices.

Prescription drugs and treatments

Before you try to conceive, tell your healthcare provider if you are using any prescription drugs or treatments. Some prescription drugs are harmful to a developing fetus. For example, Accutane, an acne treatment, has been shown to cause birth defects if taken during pregnancy.

Over-the-counter drugs and medications

Likewise, you may be instructed by your healthcare provider to stop using many common, over-the-counter medications. Several pain medications contain aspirin or ibuprofen, which may be harmful to your baby. Because of their alcohol content, using some cough medicines during pregnancy can be as dangerous as drinking wine or beer. Protect your unborn baby—before you take ANY medicine, check with your healthcare provider. In addition, inform any doctor or dentist who wants to prescribe medicine for you that you're pregnant or that you're trying to conceive.

Genetic testing and counseling

Genetic testing and counseling may help identify partners who are at risk for passing on genetically carried diseases. Genetic counselors gather facts about your family's medical history and may take samples of cells from each partner's blood to test for the presence of certain defective or disease carrying genes. They provide you with information to help you make decisions. If genetic testing is needed, it should be done before you conceive. For reliable information it is important to select an accredited genetic testing and counseling service. You might want to call your local March of Dimes organization and ask them to help you locate a qualified testing and counseling service. You might talk to a genetic counselor if:

- You and your partner are related or you are over 34
- You have had repeated miscarriages
- You have a previous child with a genetic disorder
- Any of these conditions happened in either partner's family: muscular dystrophy, cystic fibrosis, Down syndrome, mental handicap, epilepsy, liver or kidney disease, bleeding disorders, anemia, congenital heart defects, dwarfism, limb abnormalities, spina bifida
- You are of African American, Jewish, or Mediterranean descent, in whom diseases such as sickle-cell anemia, Tay-Sachs, and Thalassemia are most frequently found.

Starting your family

Discontinuing contraception
Barrier methods

You can stop using barrier methods such as condoms or a diaphragm at any time you are ready to try to conceive a baby. Many couples are surprised that the woman doesn't become pregnant right away, but it is normal for it to take several months to conceive.

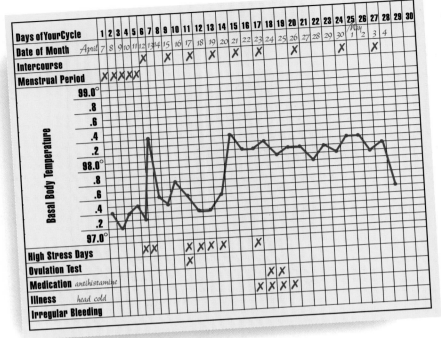

Hormonal methods

If you have been using a hormonal method of birth control, such as birth control pills, Norplant® implants, or Depo-Provera® contraceptive injections, you should use one of the barrier methods for at least one month after quitting. The purpose of this is to allow your natural hormone levels to return and to have at least one normal menstrual period before you conceive. Consult with your healthcare provider about how long you should use a barrier method—some recommend a longer wait.

Intrauterine device (IUD)

After you have had an IUD removed, you may want to have tests to be sure that you do not have a uterine infection before you try to conceive. You can use barrier methods during this time. If you become pregnant with an IUD still in place, call your nurse-midwife or physician right away. In many cases, the healthcare professional will

decide to remove the IUD as it may cause problems for you or your growing baby during pregnancy.

Predicting ovulation

In a normal menstrual cycle, your basal body temperature drops for a day and then rises just before you ovulate. By using a special basal body temperature thermometer, you can keep a daily record of changes that can help you predict when you ovulate. Just before ovulation occurs, the mucus in your vagina also becomes more plentiful and gets thinner and clearer. Ovulation predictor test kits sold at most drug stores without a prescription can help identify ovulation within 20–40 hours by a simple at-home urine test.

Keep a monthly record when you are trying to conceive. Write down all significant data, such as the information shown in the chart above. By keeping this monthly record, you will learn what is normal for your body. Take these records with you on your preconception planning visits. They will help your healthcare provider make suggestions that may help you to conceive.

Infertility

Identifying and testing for infertility

You may have had one child and suddenly find that you have trouble conceiving a second child, or you may have had children with one partner but find that you cannot conceive with a new partner. Work together as a couple to decide if you want to have infertility testing—determining that you are truly infertile and identifying the

causes can be a difficult process. You will need to reveal personal information about when and how often you make love, and the male will need to provide sperm samples.

Infertility tests are generally given over a period of months to determine what types of treatments may be recommended. Male and female infertility problems each cause about 30% of infertility cases. The remaining 40% of infertility is the result of a combination of problems in both partners or unknown causes.

Tests for male infertility may include physical examinations, semen analysis and antibody testing, scrotal and rectal ultrasound examinations, and possible testicular biopsy. Tests for female infertility may include physical examinations, basal body temperature charts, ovulation prediction tests, tests on cervical mucus taken within four hours of intercourse, laparoscopy, and endometrial biopsy. Depending on the results of each test, a specific series of treatments can be initiated. Some treatments are relatively simple, while others are complex and involve surgery for one or both partners.

Causes of male infertility

Male infertility can be caused by a number of conditions, some environmental and some a result of personal physical conditions or lifestyle choices.

- Low sperm count—Stress, illness, and infection can cause a temporary low sperm count. A varicocele, caused when blood backs up and pools in a vein in the scrotum, can block sperm.
- Blockage of the vas deferens—Sexually transmitted diseases such as gonorrhea can damage and block the normal pathway of the sperm.
- Hydrocele—Extra fluid in the testes can cause a higher temperature in the testes which can reduce sperm production.
- Ejaculation problems—Too much or too little semen often causes problems, or the semen can be very thick and can trap the sperm.

- Hormone balance—Pituitary hormones can be too high or too low.
- Antibodies—The man's own antibodies may attack and destroy his sperm.
- Chemical exposure, stress, tobacco use or secondhand smoke exposure, and alcohol use can all affect the quality and quantity of a man's sperm.
- Some illegal and prescription drugs are known to cause fertility problems.

Causes of female infertility

Female infertility can also be caused by environmental factors, personal physical conditions, or lifestyle choices.

- Ovarian problems—The ovary may not produce a mature egg. It may not release an egg due to hormonal problems or because the ovaries are scarred from previous surgery, infection, or from radiation treatments.
- Hormone balance—Menstrual hormone levels may be too low and not keep the egg alive long enough to be fertilized.
- Blocked fallopian tubes—One or both of the fallopian tubes may be blocked by tumors or damaged by sexually transmitted diseases. Pelvic inflammation resulting from pelvic inflammatory disease (PID) can block the fallopian tubes. A previous ectopic pregnancy (one in which a fertilized egg implants in a fallopian tube or somewhere other than the uterus) can also cause tubal blockage.
- Uterine problems—The uterus may have an abnormal shape or have fibroid tumors, scars, or polyps. Endometriosis, a condition in which endometrial tissue grows in abnormal locations, can cause infertility.
- Cervical mucus—The woman's cervical mucus may be too thick for the sperm to penetrate or there may be too little mucus.

The emotional impact of infertility

A wide range of emotions surface when a couple finds that one or both of them are infertile. Anger, shame, grief, sadness, and depression are common along with compassion and deep concern for the affected partner. In addition to their own feelings, a couple may be dealing with family and social pressures to conceive. They will need to gather a lot of information and decide how they feel about undergoing infertility testing, infertility treatments, or the use of assisted conception procedures.

An infertile couple may face serious financial, social, and emotional choices. Ultimately, they may choose to undergo treatment, adopt a child, or accept child-free living. Infertility therapists and support organizations are good resources to help couples sort out what is best for them. See the organization and reading resource sections of this book to find out where to get help.

Infertility Treatments

Today, couples with fertility problems have a variety of treatment options from which to choose. They should work with their healthcare provider to decide on a treatment plan, starting with the least invasive, least expensive options. It may take time for the treatments to result in pregnancy, and success is not a guarantee. Some procedures involve risks for both the mother and the baby, which couples should discuss with their healthcare provider before pursuing treatment. Couples should also see if their health insurance covers these procedures before they begin, as infertility treatments can be very expensive.

Many people have been successful in achieving pregnancy and have healthy children as a result of these procedures. Following are some of the infertility treatments available:

Fertility drugs are used to regulate hormones and trigger the release of more eggs per cycle, thus increasing a woman's chance of conceiving.

In **artificial insemination**, also referred to as **intrauterine insemination**, a concentrated dose of sperm is injected through a catheter into the uterus or fallopian tubes.

Assisted reproductive technologies (ART) are techniques that are usually recommended as a last resort because they are invasive and expensive. The following ART treatments are in order from most to least commonly used:

In vitro fertilization (IVF): Eggs harvested from the ovaries are fertilized with sperm in a laboratory; the resulting embryos are transplanted back into the uterus.

Gamete intrafallopian transfer (GIFT): As in IVF, eggs and sperm are harvested and mixed in a lab, but then the mixture is surgically injected into the fallopian tubes; fertilization occurs naturally inside the body.

Zygote intrafallopian transfer (ZIFT): ZIFT follows the same procedure as GIFT, but fertilization is confirmed before the eggs are placed in the fallopian tubes.

Intracytoplasmic sperm injection (ICSI): A single sperm is injected into a single egg; the resulting embryo is transplanted into the uterus.

Donor egg or embryo IVF: An egg or embryo donated by another woman is mixed with sperm and implanted in the uterus.

Surrogacy: Another woman carries a couple's embryo, or a donor embryo, to term.

Choices in childbearing

Informed consent

Choices based on knowledge: benefits, risks, and alternatives

Childbearing involves many choices that have both benefits and risks. Alternative forms of treatment may be available that you will want to know about before you make a decision. Because childbearing comes with so many choices, both partners need to take the responsibility to educate themselves well enough to make *informed* decisions. Selecting a caregiver who is willing to explain choices clearly and who is comfortable discussing your needs and desires is important. You will need to understand whether recommended procedures, tests, or treatments are absolutely necessary or if they are optional. In many cases you will be asked to give written informed consent.

To become an active participant in the decisions that can affect your baby's health:

- Discuss, understand, and make sure you are in agreement with any treatment, test, or procedure that is recommended during pregnancy or birth.
- Ask why it is needed and ask your caregiver to explain the risks and benefits of each test or procedure.
- Ask what alternative treatments might be tried, including "taking no action" or waiting a little longer before making a decision.

- Ask your care provider about the safety of the test or procedure. A few may carry risks of introducing infection or even terminating the pregnancy.
- Ask about the reliability of the results of the procedure or test.
- Ask what the procedure or treatment involves. Is it routine or a special circumstance?
- Ask if the test or procedure will be painful, and if so, will breathing exercises help you cope with the pain?
- Know what the test or procedure costs. Will your insurance cover the test or procedure?

- Know what will happen next after the procedure, test, or treatment is completed. Will more tests or procedures be needed depending upon the results?

Setting up a trusting relationship with your caregiver is one of the most important things you can do. Taking responsibility to be involved in decisions about your care is equally important.

Birth educators are also an excellent resource in helping you understand your pregnancy.

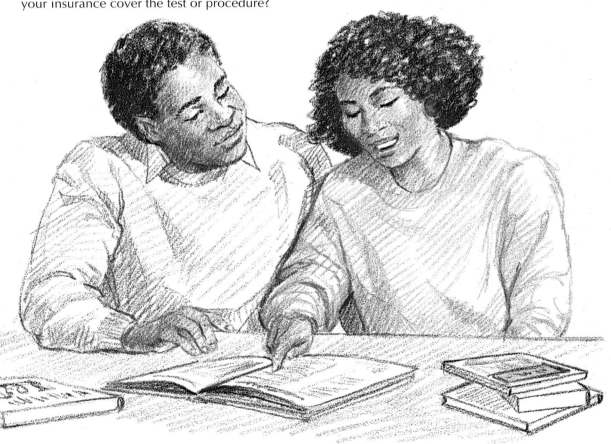

Choosing your place of birth

Before selecting a caregiver, think about your preferences for a place to give birth to your child. Most caregivers practice in only one facility, and that facility may not have all the options you prefer.

You may want to tour several hospitals and birth centers before selecting a caregiver.

Hospitals

Hospitals generally offer a medical model of care. Technology such as internal and external fetal monitoring may be used routinely even for uncomplicated labor and birth. Many hospitals now have a personal atmosphere for childbearing and offer choices in the use of technology and intervention procedures. Others are equipped to offer special care for complicated pregnancies and neonatal intensive care for babies who are born prematurely or very ill.

Freestanding birth centers

Freestanding birth centers usually practice the nurse-midwifery model of care, which embraces the family as part of the healthcare team. The atmosphere is warm and personal. Women are screened carefully during their pregnancies for any sign that they might encounter complications during pregnancy or birth. The birth center arranges for comprehensive emergency backup care with a particular hospital and physician.

> "The birth center has become a force for care—a place where families can actively decide what kind of birth experience they want to have, rather than a convenience for care providers."
>
> — **Ruth Watson Lubic, C.N.M., Ed.D.**

Birth centers or birthing rooms within hospitals

Some hospitals have a birth center or "birthing room," but these vary widely. To fully understand what your birth experience will be like in a hospital birth center or birthing room setting, ask if it is staffed by nurse-midwives or physicians, and what are the differences in procedures between the birth center and the normal labor rooms.

Home birth

In some areas, it is possible to arrange to give birth at home with the assistance of a midwife or a physician who has arranged emergency backup care with a nearby hospital.

Think about what situations make you feel comfortable. Make a list and compare how each facility makes you feel. Ask the same questions in each facility that you tour. Make notes about each facility and compare them after you have toured several facilities.

Questions to ask when choosing a birth facility

- What are the services offered for the mother and the baby?
- How much does each service cost?
- What is the philosophy of care?
- Are pregnancy and birth viewed as natural events or medical procedures?
- What educational classes does the facility offer?
- Is the staff's attitude accommodating or rigid?
- Which procedures are routine?
- Which procedures are optional?
- Will medical students or resident physicians be involved in any of your care during labor and birth?
- Can you labor, deliver, and recover in the same room?
- Does the facility have a shower or bathing facility for you to use for relaxation during labor?
- What is the facility's policy on eating or drinking during labor?
- Will you and your partner be given a time of quiet privacy after your baby is born to get to know your baby?
- What happens if the baby is born prematurely or has severe problems? Will it stay at this facility or be transferred to another?
- What percentage of births are performed by cesarean section at the facility?
- Are you free to change positions and walk during labor or will you be confined to bed or have your activity restricted?
- Are friends and family welcome to stay with you and support you during labor and birth?
- Does the facility welcome birthing assistants or doulas?
- Are siblings welcome to be part of the labor and birth if desired?

Touring the facility will tell you a lot about the attitudes and atmosphere that would surround your birth experience in each facility. Trust your instincts. You know what is best for you.

Choosing your caregiver

Once you have chosen a place to give birth you can begin selecting a caregiver. Finding someone you trust is important. You should feel comfortable having open discussions about your care. Make a list of the qualities you and your partner believe are important in a caregiver. What kind of person do you like to work with? Ask each caregiver the same questions. Make notes and use them as a checklist after you have interviewed several caregivers. Many midwives and physicians do not charge a fee for an interview visit as long as it does not include a physical evaluation. Before making an appointment, ask the office or clinic if the caregiver charges for interviews.

Like everyone else, caregivers have individual personalities. The caregiver who was right for your friend or relative may not suit you at all. The choice is a personal one, and you should not feel pressured by family members or others to go to the caregiver they chose. Your insurance plan may cover only certain hospitals or birth center facilities. They may have a list of caregivers from which you may choose. Before you become pregnant, investigate all the choices that your insurance coverage permits.

Interviewing a caregiver

Before you go, think about the type of birth experience you want and make a list of questions. You will have many questions during pregnancy and will need to know that your caregiver will take the time to listen to you with respect and answer your concerns.

Questions to consider when choosing a caregiver:

- How did the caregiver react to your questions?
- Did he or she give you clear answers?
- Did he or she ask you how you felt about a topic or view his or her opinion as the one that mattered?
- How long will he or she stay with you during your labor and birth?
- In what hospital or birth center facilities does he or she practice?
- What does the caregiver expect from you?
- What tests or procedures are routine in his or her practice?
- How often does he or she perform cesarean sections?
- Is he or she willing to discuss and honor a birth plan that you and your partner may write? Does he or she have any samples of birth plans that other couples have prepared?
- Does the caregiver practice alone or in a group?
- How does the group cover for one another?
- How does the caregiver feel about your partner or older child coming with you for your monthly checkups?
- What are the fees and payment schedules?
- What services and tests are covered by health insurance?
- Which services or tests are not covered by health insurance?
- Does the office submit insurance claims or must you pay first and then seek payment from the insurance company?
- Can the caregiver give you references for women in his or her practice who have given birth under his or her care?
- How long did it take to get an appointment?
- How long did you wait in the waiting room?
- Did the office staff make you feel welcome?
- How does the office staff treat people in person and over the phone?

Today's childbearing team

You and your partner are part of a team of professionals who share the goal of a healthy pregnancy and a healthy baby.
Preconception medicine physician
Nurse-midwife
Direct entry midwife
Obstetrician
Family medicine physician
Birth assistant / doula
Pediatrician
Birth educator
Lactation consultant

Other specialists can be called upon if needed:

Genetic counselor
Infertility counselor or physician
Assisted conception physician
Maternal / fetal medicine physician
Neonatologist

Changing caregivers

Consider changing caregivers or continuing your search if your current caregiver or the one you interviewed does not view you as a team member or listen to your concerns. There are many caregivers who will listen.

Planning for the costs of childbearing

Before you become pregnant, talk to your health insurance provider. Ask for a list of maternity and newborn services that are covered in your health plan. Ask what services are not covered.

The term "prenatal care" can mean payment for midwife or physician visits only and not cover any routine tests or diagnostic tests or treatments. Many of these tests are very expensive. Ask for a list of hospital services that are covered by insurance and those that are not covered for both mother and baby.

Other costs that you need to consider:

- Transportation to prenatal visits or facilities for special tests or procedures
- Childcare for siblings
- Prenatal vitamin prescription

- Maternity clothes
- Education classes (and transportation costs)
- Newborn clothing and layette supplies
- Diapers or diaper services
- Pediatrician fees
- Nursery furniture
- Newborn childcare if you return to work
- Loss of one income if you do not return to work

Some costs can be reduced by using equipment or clothes that friends or relatives no longer use.

Choosing the type of birth you want

Generally, pregnancy and birth are normal, healthy events. If you go to all of your prenatal visits, your caregiver can monitor your health and your baby's health for signs of complications. Most complications can be treated if they are detected early enough. As long as you are healthy, many options will be open to you concerning your pregnancy and birth experience.

There are many different philosophies and approaches to birth. Some types of facilities offer care that is more cost-efficient than others. Some will simply suit you more than others. To understand your options, talk to a childbirth educator, your caregiver, or parents who have given birth in various settings. Several excellent books are available on this subject. (See resource section.)

High-tech birth
Medical equipment and procedures have been developed for monitoring both the mother and baby in high-risk pregnancies to provide every chance for a safe delivery. Some of these procedures, such as fetal monitoring, have also become widely used in uncomplicated births. However, health professionals disagree on how much

technology should be used in a normal birth. Studies do not necessarily show better results from the use of technology in uncomplicated births. Many procedures restrict the mother's ability to move during labor. Some procedures and interventions are being linked to the rise in the cesarean section rate. Ask your caregiver what technology you can expect in your birth experience.

Gentle birth
Many health professionals believe that an atmosphere of peace and serenity can and should surround normal birth. They observe that women labor more effectively and babies adapt to life outside the womb more easily in a more natural environment. Such birth experiences can be created in freestanding birth centers, at home, and in some hospitals. Women are encouraged to move about freely during labor, choose a comfortable position, take warm baths for relaxation, and in some places to give birth in a warm tub of water if they choose. Studies have shown that in uncomplicated pregnancies the gentle birth approach is just as safe as a high-tech birth for both the mother and the baby.

Choosing who will stay with you during birth

Your partner, a friend, or a relative
Having the support and presence of a loved one has a positive effect on the progress of a woman's labor. Fathers now take active roles in learning about pregnancy and birth, supporting their partner during labor, and sharing the life-changing moment when their child enters the world. If you know in advance that the father cannot be present during labor and delivery, then choose a relative or close friend who is willing to get involved in your pregnancy, attend birth preparation classes with you, and stay with you throughout your labor and birth.

No woman should labor alone, yet many women mistakenly believe that their physician will be with them throughout their labor. In the traditional medical model of care, the management of your labor is handled by hospital staff who communicate by telephone with the physician until your labor is well established. The physician will usually arrive near the time when you start to push and deliver your baby. In contrast, the nurse-midwifery model of care offers continued support throughout the birth process.

Supporting a woman in labor is an art that can be learned in childbirth preparation classes. It is essential that the support partner learn to recognize the different phases of labor. The partner should know what relief measure will be most helpful at a particular stage. Practice together so that you and your support person develop a way to communicate.

Birth assistants and doulas

Even when a woman is prepared for birth, she may still feel anxious about being in the hospital setting with so many strangers. Hospital nursing personnel change shifts two or three times a day, and an unfamiliar physician may be on call when she is there. The general intensity of the typical hospital setting has led many couples to seek the services of a trained birth assistant or a doula (a Greek word meaning "in the service of"). A doula is usually a woman with years of experience from hundreds of births as well as professional training. Such a person gets to know the parents before birth and stays with them throughout their labor and birth experience.

A doula or birth assistant helps the parents understand what is happening during labor and suggests ways that the mother may feel more comfortable. She also serves as an advocate for the couple if the need arises. Some doulas offer follow-up services at home to help the new family get off to a good start. Studies have shown that women who are attended by a birth assistant or doula work well with labor, have positive birth experiences, and adjust to mothering more easily. A doula does not replace the role of the partner. She brings experience and perspective to help a couple have an optimum birth experience.

Choices in your labor and birth experience

Identify what is important to you during your labor and birth experience and begin writing a birth plan that will help you and your caregiver create the best experience for you. It takes a lot of conversation about choices and alternatives, and it takes time to complete your birth plan. Start to work on one early in your pregnancy.

- **Identify your concerns.** What worries you? What makes you comfortable? What is unacceptable?
- **Gather information.** What topics do you need to know more about before making your decisions? Where can you get information? Books? Educators? Caregivers?
- **Share ideas with your partner.** On what topics do you agree and disagree? Do you have friends who have had good and bad experiences?
- **Be clear about your needs.** What things are most important to you? Think about your needs in an easy labor as well as a long, hard labor or a cesarean delivery. Think about how you want to welcome your baby into the world.
- **Write your birth plan.** Follow the suggestions for creating a birth plan to help you organize your ideas and make it easier to discuss them with your caregiver.
- **Take it to your caregiver.** Communicate clearly. Discuss your needs. Listen to his or her suggestions and ideas.
- **Negotiate and come to an agreement.** Ask your caregiver to sign the plan. Request that a copy of it be attached to your medical records when they are sent to the birth center or hospital. Keep a copy for yourself.

Organizing your birth plan

Write an introductory paragraph. Describe yourself, your values, and your beliefs about the kind of birth you would like to have under the best of circumstances. Organize and list your preferences.

Birth attendants
Who will be with you? Partner, friend, or family member? Birth assistant or doula?

Early labor procedures
Do you prefer to have an enema? Do you want to have your pubic area shaved? What are your other preferences?

Positions for labor
What positions would you like to be able to use during labor—walking, squatting, or sitting? A combination?

Labor coping techniques
Would you like to be able to take a shower or a tub bath?

Medical procedures in labor
How do you feel about being able to eat or drink during labor? What about the use of intravenous fluids or the artificial rupture of amniotic membranes?

Medications
What medication options do you prefer?

Use of technology
How do you feel about the use of fetal monitoring, forceps, or vacuum extractors?

Positions for birth
What positions would you like to use while giving birth (for example, side lying or squatting)?

Medical procedures in birth
How do you feel about having an episiotomy or having your legs placed in stirrups?

Early infant contact and care
Do you want to have your baby placed on your abdomen right after birth? Do you want to breastfeed immediately?

Unexpected problems
What are your preferences in a cesarean delivery? A preterm birth? What if your baby needs neonatal intensive care?

Postpartum care and discharge
Can your baby stay with you? How long will you stay?

Care for your baby
How soon after birth can you hold your baby? If you have a boy, what about circumcision? Do you plan to breastfeed? What about bottles of water or formula?

Be flexible once you have written your plan. Labor and birth involve surprises for everyone. No two labors are exactly alike. As you approach your birth experience, know that you have done your best to define your needs and strong preferences by writing your birth plan.

Choosing pregnancy and birth education classes

Pregnancy and birth education classes are an important part of informing yourself and identifying all the options you have to consider. You will meet other expectant parents and learn how they are coping with pregnancy and the expected birth. Many classes offer a tour through the birth center or hospital. This can be especially valuable in putting yourself at ease in the surroundings in which you will give birth. Ask your caregiver and friends or check your local phone directory to see if any of the following types of childbearing classes are available in your community:
• Prepregnancy planning
• Pregnancy exercise
• Early pregnancy
• Pregnancy nutrition
• Pregnancy relaxation and massage
• Labor and birth preparation
• Siblings and birth
• Parenting and baby care
• Grandparenting
• Breastfeeding
• Cesarean delivery
• Vaginal birth after cesarean (VBAC)

Genetics and reproduction

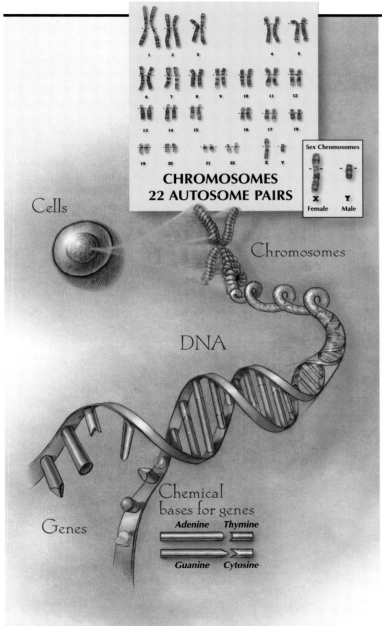

Cells

Chromosomes

DNA

Genes

**CHROMOSOMES
22 AUTOSOME PAIRS**

Sex Chromosomes

X
Female

Y
Male

Chemical
bases for genes

Adenine   Thymine

Guanine   Cytosine

Understanding basic genetics

Most of our cells have a nucleus. The nucleus contains chromosomes. Chromosomes are made up of strands of deoxyribonucleic acid (DNA). DNA strands carry a series of chemical base pairs that form genes. Genes carry all of our hereditary material and determine nearly everything about how we look, how we grow, how we function, and in some cases what diseases we will have. Today, childbearing couples need to have an understanding of what genes are, where genes are found, and how genetics may affect their child.

Cells

Every nucleus contains 23 pairs of chromosomes. There are 22 pairs called autosomes and one pair of sex chromosomes, the X or Y chromosomes. The sex chromosomes determine whether we are male or female. Our reproductive cells are unique because they carry only one half of the 22 autosome pairs of chromosomes and either the X or the Y sex chromosome. A single sperm (the male reproductive cell) contains either a single X or a single Y sex chromosome. An egg or ovum (the female reproductive cell) always contains a single X chromosome.

Almost every cell in the body contains about 200,000 genes. The genes are divided among the 23 chromosome pairs. Genes are arranged in series within DNA and are found in the same order in every human.

Chromosomes and cell division

Chromosomes are made up of DNA. It is possible to identify each of the chromosomes in early cell division when they coil tightly and thicken. Part of the process of cell division involves making a copy of the DNA (replication) so that each new cell that forms will have the same genetic information.

DNA

The DNA ladder consists of two molecular chains twisting and spiraling to form a double helix. The sides of the DNA ladder are made up of alternating phosphate and deoxyribose sugar molecules. The rungs of the ladder contain complementary base pairs arranged in any order along the DNA strand. It takes at least 10 base pairs to form one complete turn of the DNA helix.

Genes

Genes are arranged in a line along each strand of the DNA helix. The building block of a gene is a series of any three of four chemical bases. A simple gene may combine only a few building blocks and carry out simple functions. Complex genes combine hundreds or thousands of building blocks and direct very complicated functions.

Genes determine nearly everything about a person. Each gene is either dominant or recessive. A dominant gene, like the one for brown hair, is always expressed even if it is only present in one chromosome of a chromosome pair.

Nucleotide

The base unit of a nucleic acid is called a nucleotide. Its "backbone" is made of one phosphate and one deoxyribose sugar. The sugar connects to one of four chemical bases that are bonded by hydrogen into complementary base pairs.

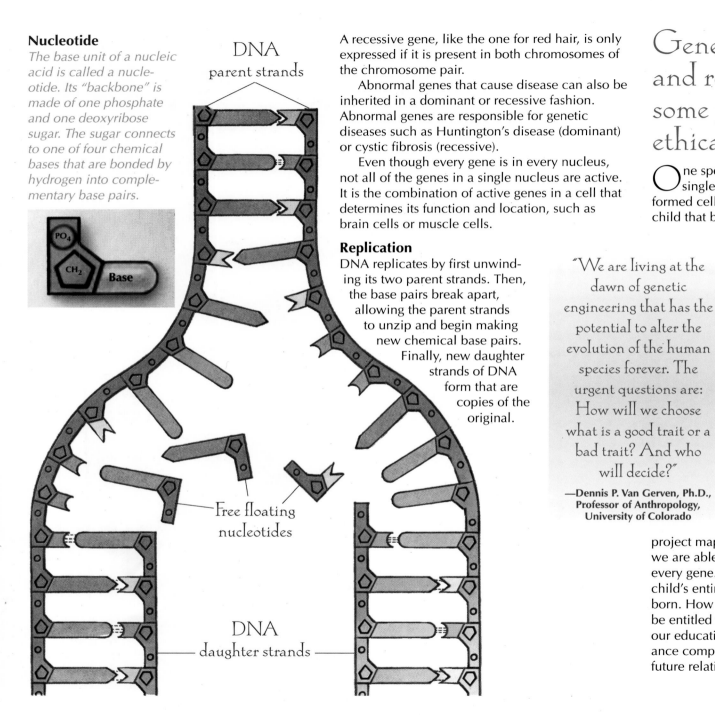

DNA
parent strands

PO₄

CH₂   Base

Free floating
nucleotides

DNA
daughter strands

A recessive gene, like the one for red hair, is only expressed if it is present in both chromosomes of the chromosome pair.

Abnormal genes that cause disease can also be inherited in a dominant or recessive fashion. Abnormal genes are responsible for genetic diseases such as Huntington's disease (dominant) or cystic fibrosis (recessive).

Even though every gene is in every nucleus, not all of the genes in a single nucleus are active. It is the combination of active genes in a cell that determines its function and location, such as brain cells or muscle cells.

Replication

DNA replicates by first unwinding its two parent strands. Then, the base pairs break apart, allowing the parent strands to unzip and begin making new chemical base pairs. Finally, new daughter strands of DNA form that are copies of the original.

> "We are living at the dawn of genetic engineering that has the potential to alter the evolution of the human species forever. The urgent questions are: How will we choose what is a good trait or a bad trait? And who will decide?"
>
> **—Dennis P. Van Gerven, Ph.D., Professor of Anthropology, University of Colorado**

Genetic technology and reproduction: some practical and ethical questions

One sperm and one ovum join to create a single new cell at conception. The newly formed cell divides again and again. At birth, the child that began as a single cell will have several trillion cells. Half of the child's genes come from the mother and half from the father. It is this unique mix of genes that makes each human being different.

Reproductive genetic technology and engineering are growing at an astounding rate. In the near future, childbearing women and their partners will face many decisions regarding the use of this technology. How will we use the information and the technical skills that are rapidly advancing? How will we weigh the potential for beneficial or harmful uses of new genetic technology? Who will determine what is ethical and unethical?

As the Human Genome project maps the location of every human gene, we are able to find out more about the function of every gene. Soon, we will be able to read a child's entire genetic blueprint even before he is born. How will we use this information? Who will be entitled to have access to this information—our education systems, our health and life insurance companies, our potential employers, or future relatives?

Genetic engineering will make it possible to decide many things about our unborn children—including their gender, personal appearance, or personality traits. What values will we assign to any given trait? Will we have a choice in the use of genetic technology?

Know your family medical history

Your family has its own genetic history, which has been passed on from generation to generation. Your partner's family also has its own unique pool of genes. Life-threatening diseases can be passed through families in the same way that physical traits such as size and eye color are passed. A disease-causing gene may exist in a family member and not cause a condition or trait for several generations. However, it may be passed on to a later generation, where it will become active. Both partners should ask family members about any diseases within the family and try to find out how relatives in past generations died. Keeping a written record of this information will help your caregivers predict if your children are at risk for a genetically carried birth defect or disease.

Chromosome disorders
An error in the number of chromosomes may happen when either the egg or the sperm form or when the fertilized cell starts dividing after conception. The error results in a cell that has an extra chromosome. For instance, Down syndrome is caused by having a third or extra copy of chromosome number 21.

Genetic diseases and birth defects
Genetically linked diseases can be passed to the next generation in two ways: the egg or sperm contain a disease carrying gene, or a single gene fails to make a perfect copy of itself during cell division. A small change called a mutation is made in the structure of a single gene during the copying process. A mutation might be harmful or beneficial. It can create a life threatening disease, cause a birth defect, or possibly even offer protection against disease. If a disease-carrying mutant gene is contained in either the sperm or egg cell, it will copy itself in all of the body cells in the growing fetus. As a result, it may cause a disease or a congenital birth defect.

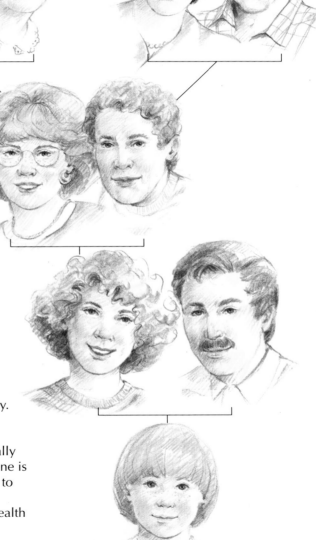

Gender-linked diseases
Muscular dystrophy is an example of a genetic disease that is caused by defective or diseased genes that are usually transmitted from one gender to the same gender in the next generation. A healthy gene from one partner can mask a defective gene contributed by the other partner. The disease will not appear in one generation and yet it can be passed on to the next.

Gene therapy
Gene therapy is sometimes called gene surgery. It is a new field of medicine that seeks to develop genetic technology that will restore health for a person who has a certain genetically linked disease. In gene therapy, a defective gene is replaced with a new gene or a gene is treated to correct the condition caused by the defective gene. Gene therapy may result in improved health for one individual but does not affect future generations—in other words, genetic material altered by gene therapy cannot be passed on.

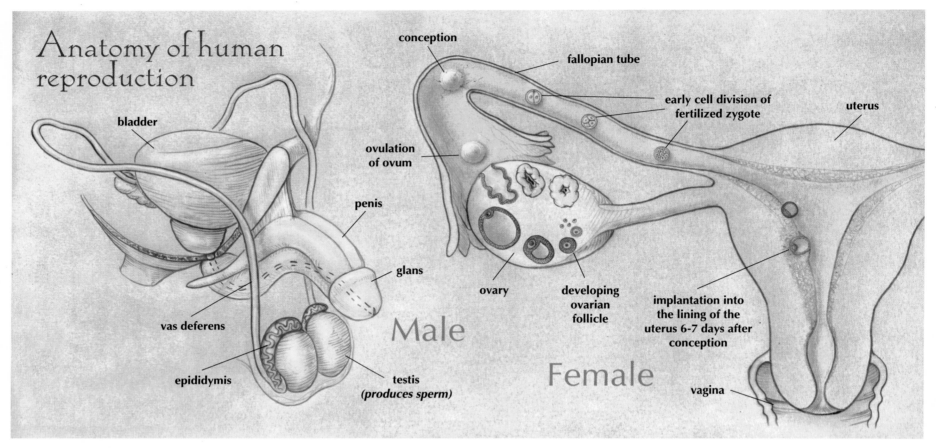

Anatomy of human reproduction

bladder

penis

glans

vas deferens

epididymis

testis
(produces sperm)

Male

conception

fallopian tube

early cell division of fertilized zygote

uterus

ovulation of ovum

ovary

developing ovarian follicle

implantation into the lining of the uterus 6-7 days after conception

vagina

Female

Conception

During sexual intercourse, the man's sperm are deposited in the woman's vagina near the opening of her cervix. The sperm travel up through the woman's uterus and into her fallopian tubes. If an egg has been released from her ovary within the past 24 hours, one of the millions of sperm may locate the waiting egg and fertilize it. This is the moment of conception.

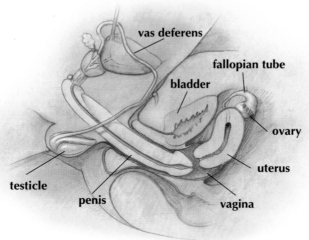

vas deferens

fallopian tube

bladder

ovary

uterus

testicle

penis

vagina

Are you having a girl or a boy?

The sex of a child is determined by its father. A man's sperm carries either an X (female) or a Y (male) chromosome. A woman's ovum (egg) always carries an X (female) chromosome. When the sperm and egg combine, the union results in either a female (XX) or a male (XY).

Girl XX
X Egg
X Sperm

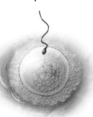

Boy XY
X Egg
Y Sperm

How twins form

Fraternal twins

Why are they different? Fraternal twins are different because they come from the union of two different eggs with two different sperm. Each egg and sperm is slightly different in genetic information, just like single-born brothers and sisters.

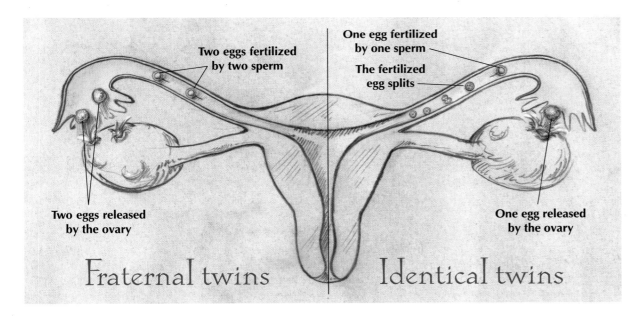

Two eggs fertilized by two sperm

One egg fertilized by one sperm

The fertilized egg splits

Two eggs released by the ovary

One egg released by the ovary

Fraternal twins   Identical twins

Identical twins

Why are they the same?
They are identical because they come from the union of one egg and one sperm that later splits into two embryos that have identical genetic information. They then grow into separate but identical babies.

Signs of pregnancy

Hormonal changes

When you conceive, your body begins to make extra estrogen and progesterone in order to maintain the pregnancy. After the 12th week of pregnancy, when it is fully developed, the placenta takes over the job of maintaining the additional levels of these hormones.

Missed period

Two weeks after conception, most women will not have their normal menstrual period. Menstruation doesn't occur because the body is preparing the uterine lining to accept a fertilized egg. The menstrual cycle will not return again until after the pregnancy.

Weariness

The energy needed to nourish a new and rapidly growing life demands a lot of your body. The uterus and placenta are growing as well. You may be especially tired in the beginning of pregnancy.

Breast changes

From the beginning of your pregnancy, hormones start to prepare your breasts for breastfeeding. Your breasts may feel full, heavy, tingly, or sore. The areola (the area around your nipple) may darken. Small bumps called Montgomery's glands develop to help lubricate your nipple and areola.

"Morning" sickness

Adjusting to rising hormone levels can cause nausea and even vomiting in some women. Many women experience morning sickness when they first get up, but it can actually occur at any time of the day or night.

Sense of smell

You may notice certain odors more or find that smoke and heavy scents bother you.

Odd taste and cravings

Increased saliva, a metallic taste in the mouth, or strange cravings are common in the early months of pregnancy. A few women even experience cravings for non-food items. Resist these cravings. These items have no nutritional value and may contain harmful substances.

Frequent urination

Your uterus is just above your bladder; as it begins to grow, it puts pressure on your bladder, making it feel as if it is full.

Heavier vaginal discharge

Hormones cause the glands in your vagina to produce more mucus than usual.

Mood swings

Changing hormone levels cause many women to experience rapid mood swings just before they have a menstrual period. The rapidly rising hormone levels of early pregnancy can have the same effect.

Pregnancy tests

Urine test

The pregnancy hormone human chorionic gonadotropin (HCG) can be found in your urine two or more weeks after conception.

Urine testing is about 90 percent reliable and can be done in an office or clinic or at home with a home test kit. Home test kits are available in the pharmacy section of many drug or grocery stores and may be used about two days after your missed period.

If you decide to use a pregnancy home test kit, be sure to follow the test's instructions exactly. If you test negative, repeat the test in about seven days to be sure that you are not pregnant.

Internal exam

About four to six weeks after conception, your physician or midwife can perform an internal exam that reveals certain signs of pregnancy. Because of increased blood volume, your cervix is softer and purplish in color. In addition, your uterus will be slightly larger and softer than usual.

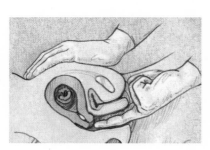

Blood test

A blood sample taken by your caregiver can detect the pregnancy hormone HCG in your blood about two weeks after conception.

Calculating your due date

This chart will help you find your due date. The date shown is based on a 28-day menstrual cycle. Pregnancy lasts 280 days or approximately 40 weeks from the first day of your last menstrual period. Remember that a due date is an estimated day of birth. Most babies are born a little before or a little after their actual "due date."

Put line under the important dates in your pregnancy.

If your last menstrual period started on:	Conception probably happened around:	All major organs are forming. Your growing baby is at greatest risk for birth defects from:		Your risk of miscarriage is less after 12 weeks:	A premature baby would have some chance to survive after:	Your estimated date of confinement (EDC) due date of conception is:
Jan 1	Jan 15	Feb 5	— Mar 12	Mar 26	Jun 11	Oct 8
Jan 8	Jan 22	Feb 12	— Mar 19	Apr 2	Jun 18	Oct 15
Jan 15	Jan 29	Feb 19	— Mar 26	Apr 9	Jun 25	Oct 22
Jan 22	Feb 5	Feb 26	— Apr 2	Apr 16	Jul 2	Oct 29
Jan 29	Feb 12	Mar 5	— Apr 9	Apr 23	Jul 9	Nov 5
Feb 5	Feb 19	Mar 12	— Apr 16	Apr 30	Jul 16	Nov 12
Feb 12	Feb 26	Mar 19	— Apr 23	May 7	Jul 23	Nov 19
Feb 19	Mar 5	Mar 26	— Apr 30	May 14	Jul 30	Nov 26
Feb 26	Mar 12	Apr 2	— May 7	May 21	Aug 6	Dec 3
Mar 5	Mar 19	Apr 9	— May 14	May 28	Aug 13	Dec 10
Mar 12	Mar 26	Apr 16	— May 21	Jun 4	Aug 20	Dec 17
Mar 19	Apr 2	Apr 23	— May 28	Jun 11	Aug 27	Dec 24
Mar 26	Apr 9	Apr 30	— Jun 4	Jun 18	Sep 3	Dec 31
Apr 2	Apr 16	May 7	— Jun 11	Jun 25	Sep 10	Jan 7
Apr 9	Apr 23	May 14	— Jun 18	Jul 2	Sep 17	Jan 14
Apr 16	Apr 30	May 21	— Jun 25	Jul 9	Sep 24	Jan 21
Apr 23	May 7	May 28	— Jul 2	Jul 16	Oct 1	Jan 28
Apr 30	May 14	Jun 4	— Jul 9	Jul 23	Oct 8	Feb 4
May 7	May 21	Jun 11	— Jul 16	Jul 30	Oct 15	Feb 11
May 14	May 28	Jun 18	— Jul 23	Aug 6	Oct 22	Feb 18
May 21	Jun 4	Jun 25	— Jul 30	Aug 13	Oct 29	Feb 25
May 28	Jun 11	Jul 2	— Aug 6	Aug 20	Nov 5	Mar 4
Jun 4	Jun 18	Jul 9	— Aug 13	Aug 27	Nov 12	Mar 11
Jun 11	Jun 25	Jul 16	— Aug 20	Sep 3	Nov 19	Mar 18
Jun 18	Jul 2	Jul 23	— Aug 27	Sep 10	Nov 26	Mar 25
Jun 25	Jul 9	Jul 30	— Sep 3	Sep 17	Dec 3	Apr 1
Jul 2	Jul 16	Aug 6	— Sep 10	Sep 24	Dec 10	Apr 8
Jul 9	Jul 23	Aug 13	— Sep 17	Oct 1	Dec 17	Apr 15
Jul 16	Jul 30	Aug 20	— Sep 24	Oct 8	Dec 24	Apr 22
Jul 23	Aug 6	Aug 27	— Oct 1	Oct 15	Dec 31	Apr 29
Jul 30	Aug 13	Sep 3	— Oct 8	Oct 22	Jan 7	May 6
Aug 6	Aug 20	Sep 10	— Oct 15	Oct 29	Jan 14	May 13
Aug 13	Aug 27	Sep 17	— Oct 22	Nov 5	Jan 21	May 20
Aug 20	Sep 3	Sep 24	— Oct 29	Nov 12	Jan 28	May 27
Aug 27	Sep 10	Oct 1	— Nov 5	Nov 19	Feb 4	Jun 3
Sep 3	Sep 17	Oct 8	— Nov 12	Nov 26	Feb 11	Jun 10
Sep 10	Sep 24	Oct 15	— Nov 19	Dec 3	Feb 18	Jun 17
Sep 17	Oct 1	Oct 22	— Nov 26	Dec 10	Feb 25	Jun 24
Sep 24	Oct 8	Oct 29	— Dec 3	Dec 17	Mar 4	Jul 1
Oct 1	Oct 15	Nov 5	— Dec 10	Dec 24	Mar 11	Jul 8
Oct 8	Oct 22	Nov 12	— Dec 17	Dec 31	Mar 18	Jul 15
Oct 15	Oct 29	Nov 19	— Dec 24	Jan 7	Mar 25	Jul 22
Oct 22	Nov 5	Nov 26	— Dec 31	Jan 14	Apr 1	Jul 29
Oct 29	Nov 12	Dec 3	— Jan 7	Jan 21	Apr 8	Aug 5
Nov 5	Nov 19	Dec 10	— Jan 14	Jan 28	Apr 15	Aug 12
Nov 12	Nov 26	Dec 17	— Jan 21	Feb 4	Apr 22	Aug 19
Nov 19	Dec 3	Dec 24	— Jan 28	Feb 11	Apr 29	Aug 26
Nov 26	Dec 10	Dec 31	— Feb 4	Feb 18	May 6	Sep 2
Dec 3	Dec 17	Jan 7	— Feb 11	Feb 25	May 13	Sep 9
Dec 10	Dec 24	Jan 14	— Feb 18	Mar 4	May 20	Sep 16
Dec 17	Dec 31	Jan 21	— Feb 25	Mar 11	May 27	Sep 23
Dec 24	Jan 7	Jan 28	— Mar 4	Mar 18	Jun 3	Sep 30

1	O
2	N
3	E
4	
5	T
6	W
7	O
8	
9	T
10	H
11	R
12	E E
13	F
14	O
15	U
16	R
17	F
18	I
19	V
20	E
21	S
22	I
23	X
24	
25	S
26	E
27	V E N
28	
29	E
30	I
31	G
32	H
33	T
34	N
35	I
36	N E
37	T
38	E
39	N
40	
41	
42	

FIRST TRIMESTER · SECOND TRIMESTER · THIRD TRIMESTER

Weeks   Months are shown in 28 day "lunar" months

1 Month

The developing pregnancy

Blastocyst – Embryo

- The fertilized egg (zygote) divides again and again, forming a ball of cells. Inside the ball, three separate layers form. Each layer has a special function that will develop and create your unique baby.
- All major organs begin to form by the end of the first month. A yolk sac develops to supply blood cells to the blastocyst until the liver and heart can develop enough to take over.
- Weight at one month: less than 1 ounce

Father

- Pregnancy may feel like a shock at first, even if it was planned.
- You may feel joy and pride along with disbelief.
- You may be surprised by the mother's mood swings and concerned about her fatigue and nausea.

Mother

- You miss your menstrual period and confirm your pregnancy with a test.
- You may feel tired, have tender breasts, and urinate frequently. You may feel nauseated.

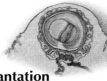

Conception

Early cell division

Implantation

- Pregnancy hormones may cause mood swings.
- If you are not already taking prenatal vitamins, see your caregiver and start taking them as early in your pregnancy as possible. The extra folic acid and iron can help reduce the risk of certain birth defects of the spine and brain.

Uterus

- The blood supply to the uterus increases to create a thick, soft lining to nourish the fertilized egg (zygote) as it implants.
- The cervix and uterus become softer.
- By the end of the first month, tiny finger-like projections called chorionic villi surround the ball of cells and help it attach to the lining of the uterus.

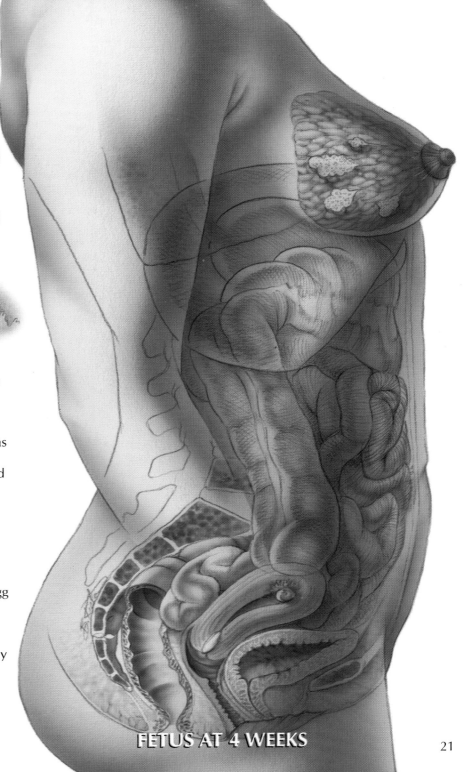

FETUS AT 4 WEEKS

Adjusting to pregnancy

Taking care of yourself

You will notice that your hair, skin, and teeth need extra care. Your body is putting so much energy into nurturing a baby that it may neglect its own needs. Resting during the day helps your body replace its energy reserves. Put your feet up and take several short breaks or a nap during your day. Avoid contact with adults or children who have a high fever or who are ill. Ask your caregiver before taking any medication or getting any vaccinations while you are pregnant. Some can damage a growing fetus.

Single mothers

Single mothers have the additional challenge of coping with the responsibilities of childrearing without daily help from a partner. You may feel social pressures, whether you are pregnant by choice or by chance. Assemble a network of strong support from family, friends, and health professionals who will help you throughout your pregnancy. Find a friend who can stay with you throughout your labor and birth. Ask your caregiver how you can contact a birth assistant or doula who can help you both during labor and the early weeks with your newborn. Your local health department may be able to provide a list of community resources for pregnant women and new mothers. Try to join a new mother's support group while you are pregnant. They offer assistance to all new mothers adjusting to parenting and provide a network of friends who help each other to grow as new parents.

Pregnancy and your workplace

If you are exposed to hazardous materials or secondhand smoke where you work, you should request a change in your job during your pregnancy. If you do work that requires heavy lifting, ask to be assigned different duties—heavy lifting is not recommended during pregnancy as it can result in strain and injury.

Think about what you need in terms of a flexible schedule, time off for prenatal care, and a place to store healthy snacks and to take short breaks in your day. Talk with your employer. Put your needs and requests in writing and ask for a copy of the company's maternity leave policy. Decide when you want to stop working and when (or if) you want to return. When you discuss your pregnancy with your employer, emphasize that you are still committed to doing your job well and that the changes or adjustments you are requesting are designed to help you have a healthy, full-term pregnancy and a healthy baby. A mother and baby who are healthy will result in lower insurance costs and fewer work days missed.

How to handle "advice"

As soon as you announce your pregnancy, it seems that everyone you meet has to tell you an old wives' tale, relate a birth horror story, or give you "advice" on what you should do or should not do while you are pregnant. Sometimes these comments can leave you frightened or wondering about your pregnancy and your baby. Don't take any of these comments too seriously. Trust yourself. You know your body and your baby. Talk it over with your caregiver if you are truly worried about anything you hear.

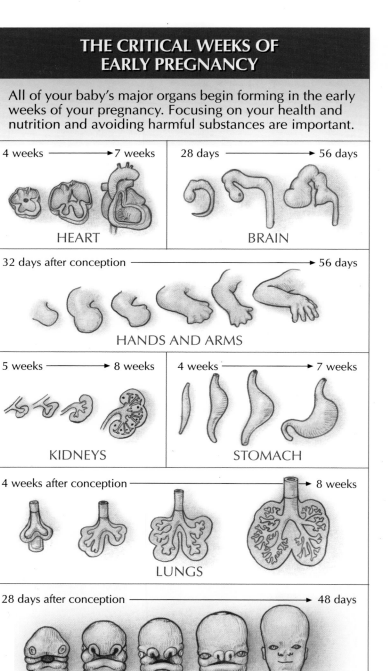

THE CRITICAL WEEKS OF EARLY PREGNANCY

All of your baby's major organs begin forming in the early weeks of your pregnancy. Focusing on your health and nutrition and avoiding harmful substances are important.

4 weeks → 7 weeks
HEART

28 days → 56 days
BRAIN

32 days after conception → 56 days
HANDS AND ARMS

5 weeks → 8 weeks
KIDNEYS

4 weeks → 7 weeks
STOMACH

4 weeks after conception → 8 weeks
LUNGS

28 days after conception → 48 days
FACE AND EYES

Environmental hazards

Hazards at home
Think about the different types of products you use on a daily basis. We take for granted the safety of many products and medicines. When you are pregnant, though, you must take special precautions to ensure the health of your baby.

Pesticides, herbicides, and fungicides
During pregnancy, take care to avoid contact with pesticides, herbicides, and other similar products. They can cause sterility, miscarriages, and birth defects.

Chemical solvents and fumes
Avoid inhaling any chemical substance that has strong vapors, especially paint thinner, turpentine, oven cleaners, or cleaning fluids.

Hot tubs, spa bathtubs, and saunas
Avoid exposing your unborn baby to the heat from very hot baths, hot tubs, spa tubs, and saunas. This heat, which is similar to your having a fever, may put your baby at risk.

Aspirin and other drugs
Do not take aspirin during pregnancy unless your caregiver has approved its use. Certain antibiotics, antihistamines, diuretics, and other drugs are known to be harmful to an unborn baby. Always ask your caregiver before taking **any** drug or medication.

Toxoplasmosis
Toxoplasmosis is caused by a parasite that infects animals; it is passed to humans through contact with animal feces. While pregnant, you should not clean a cat's litter box or expose yourself to other animal feces. Toxoplasmosis can cause miscarriage and stillbirth and can also lead to eye infections, seizures, cerebral palsy, enlarged liver and spleen, pneumonia, and mental retardation. Also avoid eating raw meat, as it can carry the parasite; wash your hands thoroughly after handling raw meat.

Lead dust
Lead, which is frequently found in exterior and interior paints used in older homes and apartments, can be harmful to the health of your baby. If you live in a house painted with lead-based paint, avoid contact with lead dust and wash your hands often.

Hazards at work
Think about where you work. While you are trying to get pregnant or during pregnancy you can put your pregnancy at risk or increase your chances of having a child with a birth defect if you expose yourself to the following:

Anesthetic gases
Exposure to anesthetic gases can cause sterility, miscarriage, and birth defects.

Dry cleaning solution
Benzene vapors released by dry cleaning solvents can cause chromosome mutations.

Other chemicals
Change your job if your work exposes you to mercury, cadmium, lead, ozone, formaldehyde, boron, manganese, PCB, PBB, carbon monoxide, rubber, or vinyl. Exposure to these chemicals can be harmful to your unborn baby.

Radiation
Both you and your partner should avoid radiation exposure while trying to conceive. While pregnant, you should avoid exposure to radiation, as it can cause birth defects.

Lifting
Your back supports nearly the entire weight of the uterus. If your job involves heavy lifting, you may need to change your responsibilities during pregnancy.

Pregnancy loss

Warning signs of miscarriage
Several signs warn of possible miscarriage. Call your caregiver right away if you have any of the following:
- Vaginal spotting of brown blood or bleeding of any amount
- Cramping in the abdomen
- Fever, dizziness, or fainting
- Severe headache, nausea, or vomiting
- Swollen joints or severe backache
- Sudden loss of pregnancy symptoms

Your caregiver will probably want to do a pelvic exam, test your blood for the HCG pregnancy hormone, and perhaps do an ultrasound scan. Here is what you can do: get off your feet and get as much rest as you can for 24 to 48 hours. Lying on your left side will help increase the blood flow to your uterus and baby. Report any increasing symptoms to your caregiver.

If you miscarry or have a stillbirth
From a medical viewpoint, if a pregnancy ends before the 22nd week it is called a miscarriage. After that point it is considered a stillbirth. If a baby dies while it is still in the uterus, labor will usually start within two to three days. The mother will need the same support as she would for any labor. Whether it is a miscarriage or a stillbirth, to the parents it is the loss of their dreams, their child. The loss is more than physical; it is intensely emotional. Friends and family may not understand the deep bond that can be formed with an unborn child no matter how early in pregnancy the loss occurs. Ask your local librarian to help locate one of the organizations of families who have lost a child during pregnancy. Such organizations have members who have experienced pregnancy loss themselves and can help other fathers and mothers deal with their grief and pain.

Dangers for you and your baby

Domestic violence

No one should ever have to endure being hit, slapped, kicked, or physically injured by any other person. Unfortunately, pregnancy sometimes triggers violence in a partner or family member of a pregnant woman. If you are being abused or are in danger of being abused, ask your friends, healthcare provider, or other people in your community for help. Talk to someone immediately if you can answer yes to any of the following questions:

Within the last year:

- Have you had threats of abuse, including the use of a weapon?
- Has anyone forced you to have sex or perform sexual acts?
- Has anyone hit, slapped, or pushed you?
- Has anyone punched, kicked, bruised, or cut you?
- Have you been beaten or sustained cuts, burns, or broken bones?
- Has anyone deliberately injured your head, back, or belly?
- Do you have any long-lasting pain caused by another person?
- Has anyone used any kind of weapon to hurt you?

Act now; don't wait to see if it happens again. Your life or your health can be in danger and so can your baby's. There are many people who will understand. Find help to protect yourself and your unborn baby.

HIV and AIDS

A woman who has HIV, the virus that leads to AIDS, can pass the virus to her baby before birth, during birth, or after birth through breastfeeding. HIV can lead to immune system damage and death. There is, however, good news for women who have HIV. Advances in HIV/AIDS treatments can help to prevent the babies of women with HIV from being infected or harmed by the virus. The sooner a pregnant woman seeks treatment, the better her baby's chances of getting some protection against HIV.

Fetal alcohol syndrome

There is no safe level of alcohol consumption if you are pregnant. Alcohol can cause fetal alcohol syndrome (FAS) or fetal alcohol effects (FAE). FAS is characterized by growth retardation, facial abnormalities, and central nervous system dysfunction. Children with FAS often display learning disabilities and serious behavioral problems. FAE refers to alcohol-related birth defects and neurodevelopmental disorders that include some but not all of the abnormalities seen in FAS babies. Children with FAE may have some of the physical or mental birth defects associated with FAS.

Experts do not know exactly how much alcohol it takes to cause damage to an unborn baby. They do know that alcohol does damage, potentially serious damage, to fetuses. Drinking alcohol during pregnancy increases the risk of miscarriage, low birthweight, stillbirth, and death in early infancy. The ability of a couple to conceive a baby can be affected by alcohol use; a man may experience lowered sperm count, making it difficult for his partner to conceive. Why take chances with your child's future? Do the best thing—avoid all alcohol while you are pregnant.

Alcohol use also affects the physical safety of both mother and child—it is a factor in a majority of accidents and violent incidents in the home.

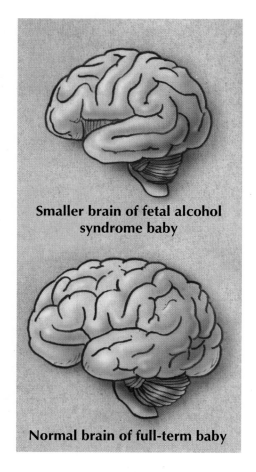

Smaller brain of fetal alcohol syndrome baby

Normal brain of full-term baby

Alcohol and the Breastfeeding Mother

Like many other harmful substances, any alcohol you drink passes into your breastmilk. Large amounts of alcohol can harm your baby. While he does not receive as much alcohol when nursing as when in the womb, alcohol still enters his bloodstream. Alcohol can also interfere with the let-down reflex (a sudden release of milk from the breast in response to stimulation), making nursing more difficult for baby and mother.

Protect your growing baby

Say NO, for your baby

Radiation and magnetic imaging
Avoid radiation exposure, including working near irradiation processing equipment or having X-rays taken. Radiation during pregnancy can harm developing fetal tissues and cause defects. Always tell X-ray technicians that you are pregnant. Require them to shield your abdomen if an X-ray cannot be avoided.

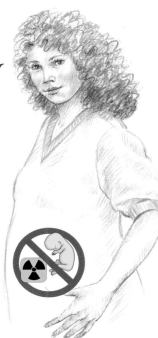

Also avoid MRI (magnetic resonance imaging), as the effects of magnetism on an unborn fetus are unknown.

Alcohol
When you drink... so does your baby. Fetal alcohol syndrome can cause major problems:
- Facial abnormalities
- Growth retardation
- Behavioral problems
- Learning disabilities

To be safe, do not drink any kind of alcohol while you are pregnant or trying to get pregnant.

Smoking or using smokeless tobacco
When you smoke or chew tobacco... so does your baby. Your unborn baby can be damaged by your smoking, by your exposure to second-hand smoke, or by your using smoke-less tobacco.
Possible results:
- Miscarriage
- Low birth-weight
- Premature birth
- Small brain size
- Early infant death
- Problems in child development

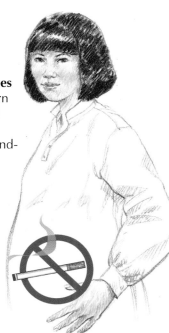

Drugs
Avoid any drug not absolutely essential to your health. Many drugs—including illegal, prescription, or over-the-counter drugs—can harm an unborn baby. Before you take **any** drug or medicine, check with your healthcare provider. In addition, inform any doctor or dentist who wants to prescribe medicine for you that you're pregnant.

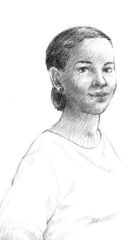

Prenatal care is important for you and your baby

Many pregnancy problems for both the mother and the baby can be treated if they are detected early. Going to all your prenatal visits helps your caregiver discover and treat possible problems before they become severe. At your first visit your caregiver will make a record of your personal health history. It will help in understanding what is normal for you. Together you can make a plan for a healthy pregnancy. Be prepared to talk about:
- Your medical history
- Your menstrual cycles
- Your family's genetic history of any major diseases
- Contraceptives used
- History of sexually transmitted diseases
- Your general health, including allergies
- Medications you have taken in the last year
- History of miscarriages or any previous pregnancies

An internal vaginal exam to check your uterus and cervix and to measure the dimensions of your pelvis will be part of this visit but probably will not be necessary at other visits until late in pregnancy.

Regular prenatal visits
If no complications arise, you will see your caregiver:
- Once a month until late pregnancy
- Twice a month during your eighth month
- Every week during your last month

Here are some of the tests you can expect at a regular visit:

- Urine test
- Weight check
- Blood pressure
- Blood sample
- Abdominal exam to measure the growth of your uterus
- Listening for fetal heart rate (FHR)
- Fetal position check/abdominal palpation

Your questions and concerns

Answering your questions is an important part of your prenatal visits. Keep a list of concerns between visits and bring them with you. No question is silly or stupid. Ask your caregiver for recommendations on books to read, and ask about pregnancy, birth education, and breastfeeding classes in your community. Ask about community support groups if you need help to quit smoking or drinking alcohol.

FIRST TRIMESTER · SECOND TRIMESTER · THIRD TRIMESTER

ONE · TWO · THREE · FOUR · FIVE · SIX · SEVEN · EIGHT · NINE · TEN

1 2 3 4 5 6 7 8 9 10 11 12 13 14 15 16 17 18 19 20 21 22 23 24 25 26 27 28 29 30 31 32 33 34 35 36 37 38 39 40 41 42

EDC · POST TERM

Weeks

Months are shown in 28 day "lunar" months

2 Months

The developing pregnancy

Five weeks

The central nervous system and all other body systems start to form at this point, although it will be months before they are fully developed. The next eight weeks are important because the embryo is very susceptible to damage.

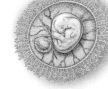

Six weeks

Amniotic fluid surrounds the tiny embryo, giving it an even temperature and protection against most infection. The face, eyes, ears, and mouth are forming and brain cells are growing rapidly.

Eight weeks

The chorionic villi burrow into the uterus and begin forming the placenta. By the end of the eighth week, your baby is one inch long, weighs less than one ounce, and is now called a fetus.

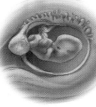

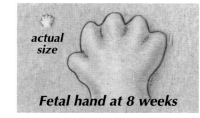

actual size

Fetal hand at 8 weeks

Father

- Worries about your changing role may begin at this time.
- Helpless feelings often arise when the mother experiences early pregnancy symptoms.
- You may be confused about how to react to rapid mood swings caused by rising hormone levels.

Mother

- Nausea may continue.
- Rising hormone levels of progesterone and estrogen can cause your emotions to be unpredictable.
- You may feel tired often and need a nap each day.
- The area around your nipples (areola) begins to darken and your breasts may feel full and tender.

Uterus

- The uterus becomes round like a tennis ball. It is still cradled within the pelvis, so most women do not look pregnant yet.
- The growing uterus puts pressure on the bladder.
- The umbilical cord develops and begins to have a definite shape and form.

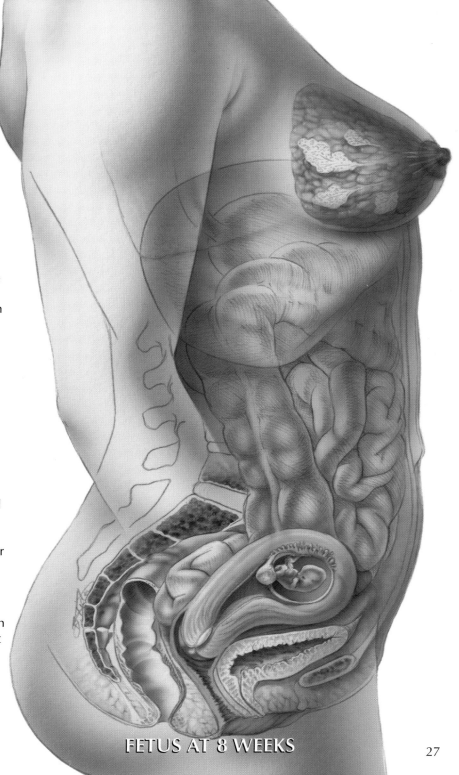

FETUS AT 8 WEEKS

27

Nurturing yourself

Becoming parents

Pregnancy often generates many fears and doubts for both partners. Such emotions are natural and are shared by all expectant parents. Pregnancy may stir desires to be cared for yourself—to be a son or daughter again. Powerful emotions often surface about how you were raised and loved by your parents. Pregnancy may be a good time for both you and your partner to examine your feelings toward your own parents and how you were raised. Communicating with your parents and dealing with these feelings now can help you define what you want to do (or not do) for your child. Resolving and letting go of conflicts from your own childhood helps you to move forward and become the parents you want to be to your child.

The mother's emotional journey

Your feelings will be greatly intensified and may be less controllable than usual during pregnancy. Emotions can range from absolute ecstasy to complete self-doubt, all due to the hormonal changes that pregnancy brings. Getting information about what is happening to your body improves your ability to cope. Many helpful books can assist you in your emotional journey through pregnancy; some of them are listed at the end of this book. Childbirth educators in your community may have a lending library of both books and videos. The public library is another good resource.

Communication is the key to resolving how you feel about your pregnancy:

- **Talk to your caregiver.** There is so much to understand about your changing body. Don't hesitate to ask any questions that you or your

"Pregnancy is a journey. At the end a woman gives birth not only to a baby, but also to her own identity as a mother."

— Gayle Peterson, Ph.D.
An Easier Childbirth

partner may have at each prenatal visit or in between visits.
- **Talk to your partner.** Talk openly with your partner about your concerns. Encourage him to share his concerns with you. Respect each other's feelings.
- **"Talk" to yourself.** Start a pregnancy journal. Write down everything you think, feel, or fear about your pregnancy, your baby, your dreams, your partner, and your changing life. Writing is one way to help you focus on what is most important to you. No one has to see the journal—it can be your private way to get in touch with how you feel on any given day.

Pregnancy and body image

Your body is already undergoing great internal change, and your body shape will also begin to change in the coming weeks. The new curves and additional weight that you will take on have a very special purpose—to nurture and protect your baby. It is normal to have fears about losing your figure during pregnancy or worry that you might never regain your figure after pregnancy. Discussing your concerns with other pregnant women or new mothers may help. If you feel overwhelmed by your fears, seek professional help.

The father's emotional journey

Expectant fathers often have many of their own fears and concerns, which they may be reluctant to express with so much focus on their partner. Fathers should talk openly and honestly about their fears, which may include:
- Queasiness about taking part in the birth
- Fears about the unknown medical establishment
- Fears about losing mother or baby

- Irrational fears about the true paternity of the baby
- Fears of being abandoned or displaced by the attention to the pregnancy or the baby
- Fears of harming the baby while making love during pregnancy
- Feelings of inadequacy or inability to help the mother cope with the stresses of pregnancy
- Concerns about handling costs of the baby
- Fears of losing independent, spontaneous lifestyle both for himself and as a couple
- Fears of assuming parental responsibilities

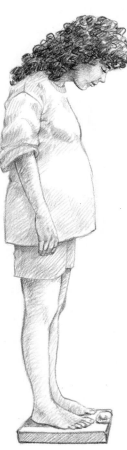

Nurturing your baby— weight gain in pregnancy

What if you are too heavy or too thin?

If you are overweight: Do not diet before or during pregnancy unless your caregiver advises you to do so. Instead, eat a balanced, nutritious diet, and avoid junk foods that are full of empty calories.
If you are underweight: You will need to gain a little more weight than average during pregnancy.

How much weight do you need to gain?

Research has proven that weight control diets in pregnancy are not good for the developing fetus. A gain of 25–35 pounds is usually considered ideal for most pregnant women. The quality of the food you eat is essential to growing a healthy baby. Eating for two does not mean eating twice as much—it means eating twice as well.

Where does the weight go?

Baby......................	7½ lb
Placenta.................	1 lb
Amniotic fluid.........	2 lb
Blood volume..........	2½ lb
Uterus....................	2 lb
Fluid in tissues........	6 lb
Breasts...................	1 lb
Fat.........................	5 lb
TOTAL...................	27 lb

How much weight will you lose at birth?
Within a few days after birth most of the weight you have gained (shaded in pink above) will be gone. Breastfeeding your baby requires many extra calories a day and will help you to lose the remaining weight more quickly.

When do you gain weight?

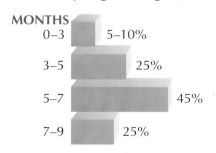

MONTHS
0–3   5–10%
3–5   25%
5–7   45%
7–9   25%

When does your baby gain weight?
In this graph, you can see that your baby gains weight slowly in the beginning and rapidly at the end of pregnancy. By the end of pregnancy, you may grow tired of thinking about what you eat and drink all the time. But your baby is still developing and depends on you to provide the nutrients to help its body grow.

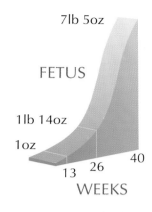

7lb 5oz

FETUS

1lb 14oz

1oz

13   26   40

WEEKS

Make healthy choices for your baby

Fats & Sweets
Use sparingly

Milk & Milk Products
4–6 servings

Fruits
2–4 servings

Meat & Meat Alternatives
3–4 servings

Vegetables
3–5 servings

Grains
6–11 servings

Nutrition During Pregnancy: Eating for Two

Nutrition is important before, during, and after pregnancy to ensure your and your baby's health. All the nutrients your baby needs while in the womb come from you and the food you choose.

Eating for two does not mean eating two times the amount of food—your recommended intake of calories is only slightly higher (by about 300 calories a day) when you are pregnant, so it is important to make wise food choices. The goal is to eat highly nutritious foods while avoiding excessive calories, fat, sugar, and sodium. Choosing nutritious foods will help lower the risk of chronic diseases and conditions such as obesity, diabetes, heart disease, high blood pressure, and osteoporosis that many women may face after pregnancy and later in life.

Your New Nutritional Needs
The following nutrients are especially important for your baby's growth and development in the womb:
- **CALORIES** for extra energy
- **PROTEIN** for your baby's new tissue growth
- **CALCIUM** for building bones
- **IRON** to develop your baby's blood
- **FOLATE** and **B VITAMINS** for cell growth
- **ZINC** for cell growth and development
- **FLUIDS** for increasing your blood supply to provide for your baby's blood supply

Exercise for a healthy pregnancy

Benefits of exercise

Being pregnant does not mean giving up all the physical activities you enjoyed before you conceived. In contrast, studies show that moderate exercise 3–4 times a week while you are pregnant:

- Increases circulation
- Increases energy level
- Eases leg cramps and backaches
- Helps to relieve constipation
- Helps to prepare your body for labor and birth
- Helps you to get your figure back sooner after delivery

Low-impact exercises like walking and no-impact exercises like swimming are best during pregnancy. Some health clubs offer special exercise programs and classes for pregnant women. If you are not normally active, consult with your healthcare provider before beginning an exercise program. All pregnant women, whether or not they exercised before their pregnancies, should avoid strenuous workouts or activities that put them in danger of falling or being hit.

General guidelines for safe exercise in pregnancy

- Always warm up before you exercise and cool down at the end of your workout.

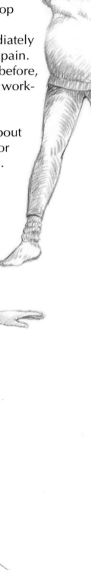

- If you get tired, begin to feel dizzy, or get too hot, stop exercising. Don't exercise if you are sick or have a fever.
- Check your pulse frequently—if it gets above 140 beats a minute, stop exercising.
- Stop exercising immediately if you experience any pain.
- Drink plenty of fluids before, during, and after your workout.
- Consult with your healthcare provider about additional guidelines or special considerations.

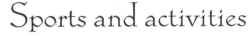

Sports and activities

Exercise, sports, and activities that involve weight burdens, bouncing or jarring motions, jumping, or sudden jerking or impact can be harmful in pregnancy.

- Jogging may be too jarring and cause your body temperature to rise too high. Brisk walking is usually a safe alternative.
- Backpacking is too stressful for your back and abdominal muscles. It's fine to go camping and hiking—just let someone else carry the gear and do the heavy lifting.
- Bicycling and cross-country skiing may be fine until you reach the point where you can lose your balance easily. Your center of gravity changes as the size and weight of your uterus increases.

Do not take part in any sports or activities that can result in a sudden impact or fall while you are pregnant, such as:

- Sky diving
- Springboard diving
- Downhill skiing
- Surfing
- Water or jet skiing
- Scuba diving
- Horseback riding
- Snowmobiling
- Rock climbing
- Motorcycling
- Ice skating
- Gymnastics

1		
2		O
3		N
4	ONE	E
5		
6		T
7		W
8	TWO	O
9		
10		T
11	THREE	H
12		R
13		E
14		E
15	FOUR	F
16		O
17		U
18		R
19	FIVE	
20		F
21		I
22		V
23	SIX	E
24		
25		S
26		I
27	SEVEN	X
28		
29		S
30		E
31	EIGHT	V
32		E
33		N
34		
35	NINE	E
36		I
37		G
38	TEN	H
39		T
40	EDC	
41		N
42	POST TERM	I

FIRST TRIMESTER · SECOND TRIMESTER · THIRD TRIMESTER

Weeks ↕ Months are shown in 28-day "lunar" months

3-4 Months

The developing pregnancy

actual size

Fetal hand at 12 weeks

Fetus

- Your developing baby is now called a fetus.
- It has teeth buds that will become baby teeth.
- The soft cartilage in the skeleton begins to change into bone. The nose begins to develop.
- The eyelids have formed and are closed firmly over the eyes.
- The external genital organs can be recognized as male or female by the end of the 12th week.
- Your baby's movements are stronger. It can roll over and open and close its mouth and fists.
- Your baby can smile and squint.
- Nails appear on fingers and toes.
- Skin is very thin and transparent.
- Your baby can hear your voice or music.
- Eyelashes and eyebrows form.
- A downy hair called lanugo covers the whole body.
- Fingerprints form.
- Your baby can swallow amniotic fluid.
- Heartbeat is growing strong and the kidneys can function.
- Weight at three months: 1 ounce
- Weight at four months: 5 ounces

Father

- Feeling helpless when the mother is sick or feeling frustrated by her mood changes is common. Remember that these changes are hormone-related and will not last forever.
- Extra financial responsibilities for prenatal care and parenthood concern many expectant parents.

Mother

- You have missed your second period. Menstruation will not return until after your baby is born.
- You may begin to gain a few pounds as the uterus, amniotic fluid, placenta, and your baby develop. Your clothes may feel tight around your waist or your breasts.
- The risk of miscarriage is very low after 12 weeks, and you may find yourself more relaxed and accepting of your pregnancy. In the fourth month, most pregnant women start to feel more energetic and have a better appetite.
- Your heart is pumping a much higher blood volume now. Almost 25% of it goes to your uterus and placenta.

Uterus

- The uterus grows to the size of a grapefruit and sits just above the pubic bone in the front of the pelvis.
- The placenta is fully formed and carries all nutrients to the baby, takes away wastes, and issues most of the hormones that maintain the pregnancy.

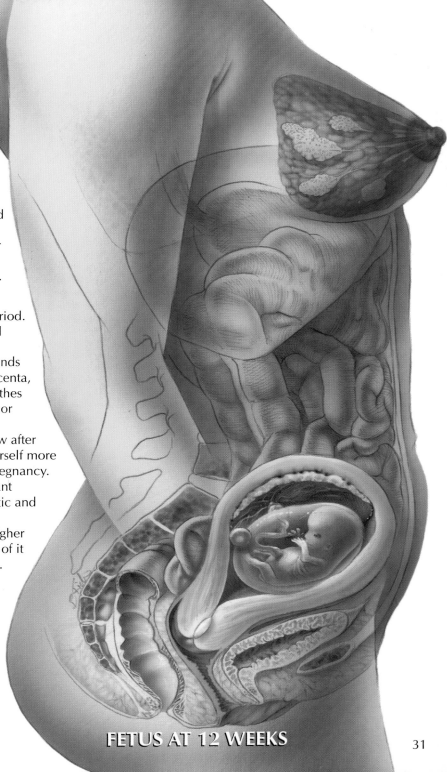

FETUS AT 12 WEEKS

31

Prenatal testing

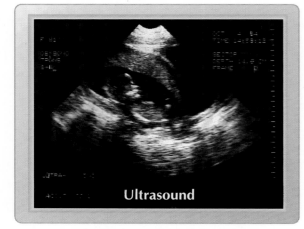

Ultrasound

Sonogram of fetus at 12 weeks

Types of ultrasound:
• Transabdominal ultrasound
• Transvaginal ultrasound
• Level II ultrasound
• Fetal echocardiography

Possible prenatal tests

Prenatal tests can help measure the growth and development of a fetus and diagnose certain birth defects. Prenatal tests do not prevent birth defects—they provide knowledge about the baby before it is born. Ask your healthcare provider about benefits and risks of each test.

Maternal serum alpha-fetoprotein (MSAFP) screening: MSAFP is a blood test used to detect a baby's risk of neural tube defects such as spina bifida, abdominal wall defects, and chromosomal abnormalities like Down syndrome. MSAFP is most often done between 15 and 18 weeks after the last menstrual period.

Chorionic villus sampling (CVS): In CVS, a sample of fetal chorionic villi is taken and used to diagnose or rule out certain birth defects. CVS is not generally offered to all pregnant women: there is some risk of miscarriage and other complications associated with the test. It is most often used in women age 35 and older, women who have had a previous child or pregnancy with a birth defect, or women and their partners who have a family history of genetic disorders. CVS is usually performed between 10 and 12 weeks after the last menstrual period.

Amniocentesis: Amniocentesis, in which a sample of amniotic fluid is taken through the uterine wall, is used when there is an increased risk of chromosomal or genetic birth defects. It can also determine fetal lung maturity. Like CVS, amniocentesis is not generally offered to all pregnant women, as there is a slight risk of miscarriage or infection. It is used for women age 35 and older, women who have had a previous child or pregnancy with a birth defect, and women and their partners who have a family history of genetic disorders. Amniocentesis is usually done between 14 and 18 weeks after the last menstrual period. It is sometimes offered earlier than 14 weeks, but the risk of miscarriage has been shown to be higher then.

Ultrasound: Ultrasound is a procedure that has many uses during pregnancy. It uses sound waves bounced off the developing fetus to create an image called a sonogram. This technique is also referred to as sonography or sonar. It can diagnose a suspected ectopic pregnancy, determine possible miscarriage, detect certain birth defects, verify due date, monitor fetal growth, diagnose multiple fetuses, and help to determine delivery method. Ultrasound can be used throughout the pregnancy.

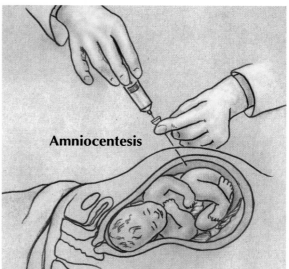

Amniocentesis

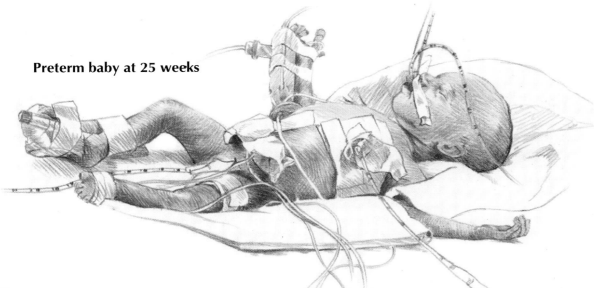

Preterm baby at 25 weeks

Prematurity is a serious problem

A baby born before 37 weeks of pregnancy or a baby weighing less than 2,500 grams (5.9 pounds) is considered a premature or preterm baby. It will need to be cared for in a Neonatal Intensive Care Unit in order to have a chance to survive. Most of a premature baby's major organs and its immune system are not mature. The baby may have problems with breathing, keeping warm, and feeding. The cost for the highly technological care that is needed ranges from $2,000 to $150,000 per infant. As premature and low birthweight babies grow up, they can have problems such as:

- Slower physical and mental development
- Special schooling needs
- Frequent illness and hospitalization
- Greater financial needs

Going to all of your prenatal visits will help you have a healthy pregnancy and avoid many of the problems that can cause preterm labor and premature birth.

Bedrest in pregnancy

Bedrest may be prescribed for women who develop problems in pregnancy or signs of preterm labor. Bedrest reduces the physical demands and stresses on your body. More energy is available to help your baby stay in your uterus and grow to "full-term" (37–40 weeks of pregnancy). Staying on bedrest can be extremely difficult, both physically and emotionally, but it may be the most important job you will ever have.

Types of bedrest in pregnancy

- Limited bedrest: You are able to be out of bed for a certain number of hours each day. You may be permitted to sit in a chair or on the sofa rather than being actually confined to bed.
- Bedrest with bathroom privileges and meals: You are required to stay in bed except to go to the bathroom and to join your family for meals.
- Bedrest with bathroom privileges: You must stay in bed, even for meals, but you may get up to go to the bathroom.
- Strict bedrest: You must stay in bed at all times

and use a bedpan rather than getting up to go to the bathroom. In some cases, you are required to stay in the hospital for close monitoring of your condition or your baby's condition.

Questions to ask your caregiver about bedrest

If you are asked to go on bedrest during your pregnancy, you will want to understand why. Ask your caregiver to explain what condition makes bedrest so important for you and your baby. You will need to establish a comfortable way of communicating with your caregiver about your progress and your baby's condition. You will also want to know:

- The number of hours of bedrest each day
- The positions that you need to use or to avoid using
- The amount of time that you can stand each day
- Any restrictions about how much weight you can lift
- Any restrictions on your sexual activity
- How to recognize and time contractions
- How to do self-palpation and kick counts
- The benefits and risks of any medications that may be prescribed to prevent preterm labor
- How long you can expect to be on bedrest
- What home care services will be provided
- What will be covered by your health insurance
- What community resources he or she can recommend
- When your caregiver wants to be called

Accepting help from family and friends

Bedrest changes your lifestyle almost overnight. It is often hard to accept help from others when you are so used to doing daily tasks for yourself. At first it may even be difficult to know what help to ask for. Start by making a list of all the things that you do each week. Think of a person who can help with each task. Friends, family, and church or synagogue members can combine some of your errands with their own and be part of your support team. Keep a list of names and phone numbers of anyone who offers to do anything for you. Don't be afraid to use it. Here are some things they might do to help:

- Shopping and running errands
- Bringing meals or helping to prepare meals
- Changing your beds or doing your laundry and house cleaning
- Taking care of any older children
- Helping you set up your "nest"

Setting up a bedrest "nest"
You will need to ask other family members and friends to help you set up your "nest." If it is possible within the type of bedrest that your care provider has ordered for you, set up two "nests" to give yourself a change of scene. Your comfort and convenience are important. Create a warm and comfortable place for yourself. Having the things you need at your fingertips will make your confinement in bed easier to tolerate.

- Turn your bed to face the window so you have a view.
- Use a portable ironing table at the side of your bed to give you extra space to keep things at hand. Adjust the height to the height of your bed. Or, buy a three-tiered rolling cart at a discount store.
- Buy an extra long (25-foot) telephone cord to put your phone within your reach.
- Keep a phone book with yellow pages near you.
- Make sure you have a reading light by your bed.
- Put a shoe bag at the side of your bed, and tuck the top under your mattress. Store items in it that you frequently use: a hairbrush, deodorant, tissues, lotion, etc.
- Get a lidded cup and use flexible straws.
- Keep a small towel handy to wipe up any spills.
- Get a home intercom system so that you can call for help if family members are out of hearing range, or use a bell or whistle.
- Use extra pillows and a bolster to support your back. You can stuff towels in a pillow case for an extra pillow and you can put tape around rolled blankets to form a bolster.
- Order an egg crate foam mattress overlay from a camping supply or a medical supply company. Staying in bed for a length of time can cause pressure points on your skin. Mattress overlays can help relieve this pressure.

Preventing preterm labor

Recognizing contractions
Although your uterus contracts normally throughout pregnancy, such contractions occur randomly and do not continue. Your uterus is more likely to contract during or after physical activity such as walking, climbing stairs, lifting, or just standing for a long time. Contractions during pregnancy feel just like any other tightened muscle. Make a fist and feel your upper arm. It feels firm and you can't press your fingertips in. When you are having a contraction your uterus will feel hard at the top, like your contracted arm muscle.

How to do self-palpation:
Feeling your uterus for contractions is called self-palpation. A wide range of contraction patterns can be considered normal. Your caregiver can help you learn what is normal for you. After the 28th week, take time to check your contraction pattern every day.

- Drink one or two glasses of water, juice, or milk.
- Urinate.
- Lie on your side. Use pillows for support.
- Put your fingertips on the top of your abdomen.
- Feel and time your contractions for one hour.
- Record how far apart your contractions were and how long each contraction lasted.

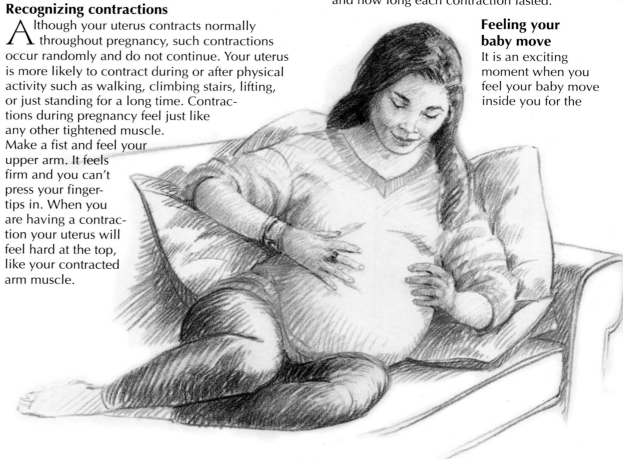

Feeling your baby move
It is an exciting moment when you feel your baby move inside you for the

34

first time. It happens around the 18th to 20th week of pregnancy and is called "quickening." Your baby has made tiny movements since the eighth week of pregnancy, but they were not strong enough for you to feel. At first it feels like "fluttering." Your baby actively kicks, moves its arms and hands, turns from side to side, and tumbles around in its watery environment.

How to count kicks

You know your baby best, and you can help track your baby's health by counting its movements once each day after 28 weeks of pregnancy. Count movements during your baby's most active time or when you do self-palpation to monitor your contraction patterns. Other times to count movements effectively might be after you drink cold water or juice, after you have eaten, or after you have walked for five minutes. Record your baby's movements.

DATE	START TIME	✓✓✓✓✓✓✓✓✓✓	END TIME
Monday 24	10:20 am		10:54 am

- Write down the time you start.
- Make a mental note (or put a check after the start time) each time your baby kicks, twists, or turns.
- After your baby has moved 10 times, write down the time again.

Some babies are more active than others even before birth. Call your caregiver if your baby moves fewer than 10 times in two to four hours or if you notice that the number of your baby's movements is slowing down.

When to call your caregiver

Call your caregiver right away if you have any of the symptoms of warning signs listed. You know your baby and your body best. Trust your instincts. Call any time you feel that something is not right.

Signs of preterm labor

- Stomach cramps: You feel cramps with or without diarrhea or vaginal bleeding.
- Contractions: You have five or more contractions in an hour. They may be painless or painful menstrual-type cramps, or a cramping feeling in your lower abdomen. The cramps may come and go or be constant.
- Pressure in your pelvis: It may feel as if your baby is pushing down. The pressure usually comes and goes.
- Low, dull backache: The pressure is usually felt below your waistline. It may come and go or be constant.
- Leaking or gushing of fluid: You feel a slow leak or a gush of fluid from your vagina.
- Change in vaginal discharge: There may be an increase in a watery, pink or brownish mucous discharge.

If you are at risk for preterm labor

- Avoid standing for long periods of time.
- Do not sit for long periods of time.
- Avoid climbing stairs.
- Do not lift children or other heavy objects.
- Ask your care provider before continuing sports or exercise.

Other warning signs

Report any of the following signs to your caregiver:
- Bleeding from the vagina, rectum, nipple, or lungs (coughing up blood)
- Swelling of the face or hands
- Severe swelling of the legs
- Severe or continuous headache
- Sudden large weight gain
- Dimmed or blurred vision, flashes of light or spots
- Chills or fever
- Severe or continuous vomiting
- Sharp or prolonged abdominal pain
- Absence of or decrease in fetal movement

Neonatal intensive care

Some hospitals and caregivers specialize in providing care to very sick and very small premature (preterm) infants. Without this help, a baby born prematurely would have very little chance of surviving outside the womb. While a preterm baby's major organs have all formed, its lungs cannot exchange air well, it is not able to maintain its body temperature, and it cannot digest its food easily. Neonatal Intensive Care Unit (NICU) staff are trained to help premature infants survive.

The best place for your baby to grow is inside your uterus. Every day, every week counts.

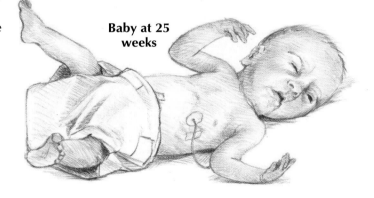

Baby at 25 weeks

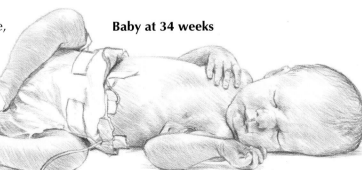

Baby at 34 weeks

New frontiers: fetal surgery

Our gains in knowledge of fetal development, genetic technology, and advances in surgical techniques have opened new possibilities. Some fetal conditions that would be life threatening if left untreated can now be corrected while the fetus is still in the uterus. Blood transfusions or medications can be given to the fetus with ultrasound guidance.

During fetal surgery, the unborn baby is temporarily removed from the uterus so that doctors can correct a condition that would prevent the unborn baby from developing normally. The fetus is then replaced in the mother's uterus to continue its development. Fetal surgery to correct defects in major organs is usually done after the 18th week of pregnancy.

1	
2	
3	ONE
4	
FIRST TRIMESTER	
5	
6	
7	TWO
8	
9	
10	
11	THREE
12	
13	
14	
15	FOUR
16	
17	
SECOND TRIMESTER	
18	
19	FIVE
20	
21	
22	
23	SIX
24	
25	
26	
27	SEVEN
28	
29	
30	
31	EIGHT
32	
THIRD TRIMESTER	
33	
34	
35	NINE
36	
37	
38	
39	TEN
40	
41	POST TERM
42	
Weeks	Months are shown in 28 day "lunar" months

5-6 Months

The developing pregnancy

Fetus
- Your baby has periods of being awake and periods of being asleep.
- It hiccups and sucks its thumb.
- Its eyes can open, close, and blink.
- The ovaries are formed in girls and contain all the eggs she will have.
- A thick coating of vernix covers and protects the baby's skin.
- The baby is active and can turn head over heels and kick.
- Weight at five months: 1/2–1 pound
- Weight at six months: 1–1 1/2 pounds

Father
- The pregnancy often becomes more enjoyable as the mother begins to feel better.
- Sexual desire may change and sexual activity and lovemaking positions may need to change as the mother's belly grows.
- You may begin to watch other parents and think about parenting styles.

Mother
- You begin to look pregnant.
- Your skin may itch as it stretches.
- You may feel sharp twinges on the sides of your belly due to the contraction of the ligaments that

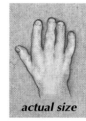

actual size

Fetal hand at 20 weeks

help support your uterus.
- You may feel leg cramps at night.
- A dark line may appear down your belly.
- Stretch marks may become noticeable.
- Dreaming at night may increase.
- Your breasts may begin to produce colostrum (the first milk).

Uterus
- At the beginning of the fifth month, the uterus is about three inches above the pubic bone. By the end of the sixth month, it will be just above the level of the navel.
- The amniotic fluid increases.
- The placenta now supplies most of the hormones that maintain the pregnancy. It also brings nutrition and oxygen to the baby and carries away wastes.

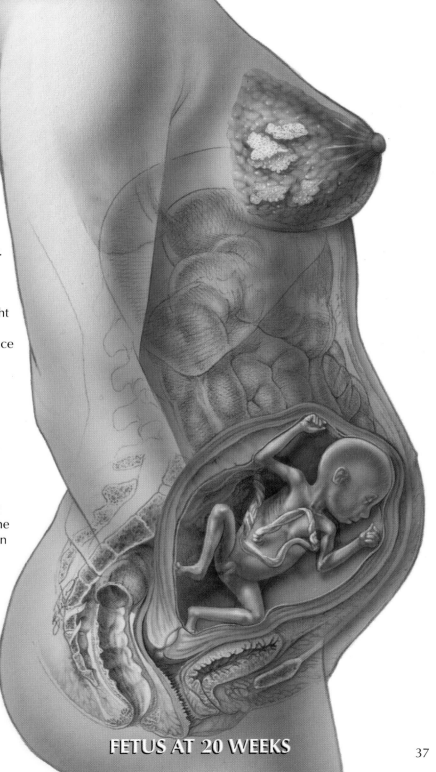

FETUS AT 20 WEEKS

37

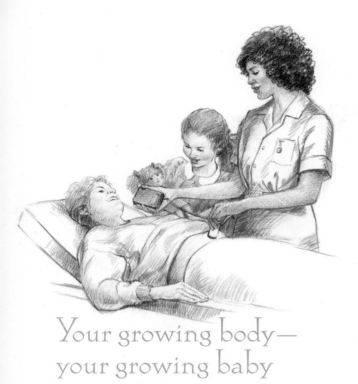

Your growing body—
your growing baby

Listening to your baby's heartbeat

An unborn baby's heart beats about 140 times a minute—almost twice the rate of an adult. Listening for fetal heart tones (FHT) is part of all your prenatal visits from about week 14 throughout your pregnancy. Your midwife or physician will use a stethoscope or a Doppler ultrasound instrument to listen. You can listen, too. Hearing your baby's heartbeat and feeling it move puts you in touch with your unborn baby in a way that nothing else can. If you bring your other children along to prenatal visits in the later months, they will delight in hearing your baby's heartbeat.

Involving your older children in your pregnancy

If this is not your first baby, you will have to decide when you are comfortable telling the older children about your pregnancy. They may not be as joyful about the idea of having a sister or brother as you might want them to be. Respect their feelings and do not try to change them. Ask your older child to draw a picture of the new baby growing inside you and to tell you about the drawing. You can make a story book together. Let the child feel your baby move. The public library or local bookstore will probably have several children's books that may help them express both their positive and negative feelings about having a new baby in the house.

Car safety

You should always wear a seat belt when driving or traveling in an automobile. Seat belt use is doubly important if you are pregnant. Seat belts and air bags are your best protection against injury to yourself and your unborn baby if you are involved in an accident. Keep the lap portion of the seat belt under your belly, low and across the pelvic area. The shoulder harness should come down over your shoulder, between your breasts, and over the top of your belly to fasten at the side. Follow your car manufacturer's recommendations for seat belt and air bag safety.

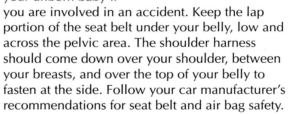

Losing your balance

Your center of gravity changes in the second and third trimesters. As your baby grows inside your uterus and your pregnancy begins to show, you will find that you can lose your balance more easily than usual. Wearing flat or low-heeled shoes or a good sports-type shoe is recommended to reduce the possibility of falling when your balance suddenly shifts.

Pregnancy & comfort

With all the activity inside your body, it's no wonder that you are probably exhausted! Weariness occurs mostly in the first and third trimesters. In the first trimester, your body is adjusting to being pregnant; the hormone changes alone can make you feel tired. During the second trimester, you may begin to feel a bit more energetic. By the end of the second trimester, your baby begins to grow and gain weight rapidly, demanding a great deal of energy from your body.

Make rest a priority during your pregnancy—getting enough rest is just as important as getting enough exercise.

Take a break and get comfortable

By now you know that growing a baby takes huge amounts of energy. Give yourself a break every day. Take the weight of your uterus off of your back and rest for half an hour. It will help to restore your energy. Gather a pile of pillows and make a pillow nest. Put pillows under your bottom and in front of you. Lean forward and relax over the pillows or use a bean bag chair.

Getting a good night's sleep

Sleeplessness can happen in all trimesters. In the early weeks of pregnancy your body is tired from increasing hormonal changes and you may not sleep well as a result. As your baby grows and begins to squirm and kick, all that activity inside you can keep you awake. The increasing size and pressure of your uterus can make it difficult to find a comfortable position. Try getting into a bedtime routine of taking a warm bath, using mild oils or creams to relieve the dryness of your stretching skin, and then fixing yourself a glass of warm milk to drink before nestling into bed.

Lying down

Lying on your side is an ideal position for either resting or sleeping. After the fifth month, if you lie flat on your back, the weight of your uterus reduces blood/oxygen flow to your baby by putting pressure on a major blood vessel along your spine. For comfort, bend your knees and elbows and use several pillows under your knees, belly, head, and back.

Getting out of bed

Getting out of bed is awkward, especially in the second and third trimesters. Take care to get out of bed slowly. In the last four or five months of pregnancy it may strain your abdominal muscles if you sit up suddenly after you have been lying down.

Follow these steps to get out of bed:
1. Roll onto your side as you bend your legs forward at your hips.
2. Swing your legs forward over the side of the bed as you use your arms to push yourself up to a sitting position.
3. Sit at the edge of the bed for just a moment, especially if you have low blood pressure. Then use the muscles in your arms and legs to push up from the edge of the bed.

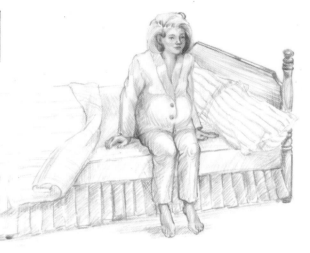

Semi-sitting

This position is sometimes preferred by women who experience nausea in early pregnancy or a lot of heartburn and indigestion in late pregnancy. For others it is a comfortable position for reading and relaxing. Prop yourself up and lean against a bolster and pillows. Put a pillow or a stack of towels under your knees to keep them flexed.

How to relieve a backache

Backache, especially lower back pain, is one of the most common complaints of pregnant women. It often includes pain across the buttocks and down the legs. Increased levels of progesterone result in softening and stretching of the pelvic bone ligaments (which will eventually allow the baby to be born). Extra strain is put on the back and hip joints. Your center of gravity also changes, which may cause your pelvis to tilt forward, putting more strain on back muscles. You may also experience some upper backache, most often limited to the first trimester, which is usually due to strain caused by rapid breast size increase.

Maintaining good posture with your pelvis tilted back will help to relieve some back pain. Try sleeping with pillows that support your legs and back, and wear low-heeled shoes. For upper back pain, a good maternity bra will usually give relief. Do abdominal exercises (with your caregiver's approval) to help strengthen the muscles that support the uterus; never lift heavy objects.

Pelvic tilt
On hands and knees
1. Get down on your hands and knees. Take care not to let your back sag downward.

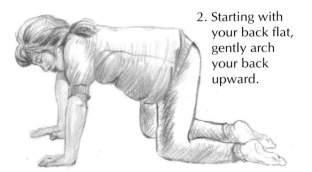

2. Starting with your back flat, gently arch your back upward.

3. Hold this position for a moment or two, and then lower your back to a flat position again. Repeat five times.

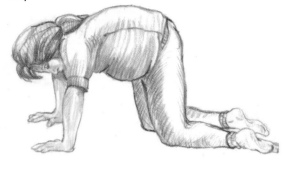

Side-lying
Lie down on your side supported by pillows. Use ice packs, a hot water bottle wrapped in a towel, or a heating pad. Hold it to the area that aches.

Standing
Lean back against a wall, and gently flatten your back to the wall by tipping your pelvis upward. Then release and repeat.

Knee to chest
This exercise relieves the tension that builds up in the back of your legs when you strain your back.
1. Lie on your back with your knees drawn up and your feet flat on the floor.
2. Slowly bring one knee up to your abdomen and hold it in that position with one hand under your thigh.
3. Pull the other leg up. Then gently and slowly pull both knees toward your shoulders until you feel a stretch in your lower back.

4. Hold this position for a count of five, and then lower your knees just enough to release the stretching sensation.
5. Repeat this motion five times, then lower your feet to the floor one at a time.

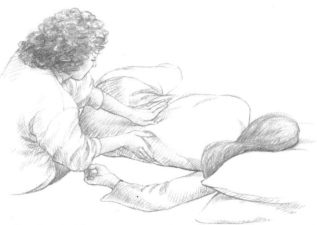

Back rubs from your partner
Getting a back rub from your partner or a friend can relieve your backache. Ask him to move his thumbs in a circle, gently rubbing your lower back. Walking his thumbs up your back while pressing gently on each side of your spine can relieve general back tension. Pregnancy is a great time to learn massage techniques that you and your partner can both use. Having your partner massage your bare back using a light massage oil to reduce friction can feel wonderful at the end of a tiring day.

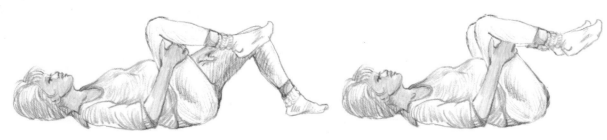

Hormones change your life

During pregnancy your levels of estrogen and progesterone will increase to nearly 10 times their normal levels. These hormones are necessary for the growth of your baby and for maintaining your pregnancy. The levels will fall sharply just after your baby is born. Your body will need about six weeks to readjust to your normal hormone levels. Hormones affect each stage differently.

Early pregnancy: Your pituitary gland, your ovaries, and your adrenal glands issue hormones that stop your menstrual cycles and prepare your body to accept the pregnancy and nourish a growing fetus. Hormones begin preparing your breasts to provide breastmilk for your newborn by increasing the size of your milk-producing glands and by starting production of colostrum, the protein-rich fluid which is produced for the first few days after birth, before your milk comes in.

Mid-to-late pregnancy: The placenta is fully formed by the beginning of your second trimester. It takes over much of the estrogen and progesterone production that maintains your pregnancy and determines fetal growth. These hormones change the function of all your major organs. They affect your skin as well. The growing fetus also produces some hormones, and it is believed that some of these fetal hormones help determine when labor begins.

Emotional swings: Your range of feelings—from absolute ecstasy to complete self-doubt—may be greatly intensified and less controllable. You may find that you get more upset about small changes in your life than you normally would and that these feelings can come on quite suddenly.

Possible skin changes: Hormones can cause itchiness, blotchy patches, rashes, and some changes in pigmentation of your skin during the second and third trimesters. Stretch marks (reddish lines

Hormones change your body

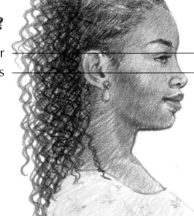

What's happening?

Eyes: cornea grows thicker
Nose: lining swells

Breasts: milk glands enlarge
Lungs: breathe more deeply
Heart: pumps 30-50% more blood volume

Metabolism: increases

Ribs: expand 2-3"
Stomach: digestion slows
Spine: supports weight of uterus

Ligaments: relax and stretch

Uterus: crowds other organs

Placenta: issues high levels of progesterone and estrogen
Bowel: functions slow

Bladder: pressured by uterus

Legs: circulation decreases

Changes in your body

Contact lenses may irritate
Nasal stuffiness, nose bleeds

Breast tenderness
Shortness of breath
Heart rate about 20% faster, blood pressure changes, dizziness, faintness

Blood sugar level change

Rib pain
Heartburn and indigestion
Backache

Sharp abdominal pain when round ligaments overstretch

Pelvic and abdominal pressure

Mood swings, insomnia, fatigue

Constipation, hemorrhoids, gas

Frequent urge to urinate, possible urinary tract infection

Varicose veins, aching legs

41

on your belly, buttocks, and breasts) appear when the underlying tissues of your skin are stretched beyond normal. After birth, they will fade and become thinner, but they will never completely disappear. A dark line from your navel to your groin may appear in the second or third trimester. You may develop more moles and freckles than you had before. You may have increased acne and sweat more than you usually do. You may also retain fluid, causing puffiness in your hands, face, and feet, especially in the last trimester.

Discomforts of pregnancy

Morning sickness
About half of all pregnant women experience some nausea and vomiting during their pregnancies. Although morning sickness is usually worse in the morning, it can strike at any time during the day or night. It usually starts between weeks 2 and 6 and ends by week 14. It isn't clear what causes morning sickness, although it is suspected to be a result of increased hormones; stress can worsen symptoms. To help combat morning sickness, eat frequent, small meals. Avoid spicy and greasy foods and foods whose smell makes you sick. Sometimes, eating crackers before getting out of bed in the morning helps, and try getting up slowly out of bed. If vomiting is severe and you can't keep fluids down, contact your healthcare provider.

Heartburn and indigestion
Heartburn is a burning sensation that can extend from the lower throat to the bottom of the breastbone. It is caused by stomach acid backing up into the esophagus. Most pregnant women experience some heartburn and indigestion during the second half of their pregnancy. Increased progesterone relaxes the valve between the stomach and esophagus. In late pregnancy, heartburn can be a

result of the growing fetus crowding the abdominal cavity. To reduce heartburn and indigestion, avoid large or high-fat meals, and avoid drinking a lot of liquid with meals; milk or yogurt may ease heartburn (unless you are lactose intolerant). Chew your food well, and stay upright for at least one hour after eating. Elevate your head when you lie down.

Constipation and hemorrhoids
Constipation results in infrequent, hard stools which can then cause or worsen hemorrhoids. It can occur throughout your pregnancy. Increased progesterone causes the intestinal wall muscles to relax, which results in more water being absorbed from the stool in the colon. The increased iron in prenatal vitamins can also lead to constipation. The best way to avoid constipation is to increase fluid intake and eat plenty of fruits (especially figs and prunes) and roughage (especially bran). Exercise regularly—squatting is especially good. Go to the bathroom as soon as you feel the urge, and avoid straining your bowels.

Leg cramps
Cramps are muscle spasms that cause a sharp pain in the thigh, calf, and/or foot followed by aching in the affected area. They usually occur in the third trimester. It is unclear what exactly causes cramps. They could be a result of the added weight and increasing pressure that the enlarging uterus is putting on the nerves and veins. Other theories are that they are caused by circulation changes or a calcium deficiency. When you get a cramp, flex your foot, bringing your toes toward you, and rub the area using firm pressure. Applying heat may also help relieve cramps. Exercise regularly, and make sure you are getting an adequate supply of calcium in your diet.

Groin pain
Groin pain happens most often in the third trimester. When the ligaments that attach your uterus to your groin are overstretched, they can contract and cause a sudden sharp pain. This can

happen when you cough, sneeze, laugh, or reach for something high above your head. Sit down until the pain is gone.

Posture and comfort
The weight of your growing uterus can contribute to backache. Look in the mirror and check your posture. Stand tall with your shoulders back and relaxed. Your back should have a comfortable curve, but avoid letting your weight shift forward and swaying your back. Keep your chin up, your bottom tucked under, and your knees slightly bent.

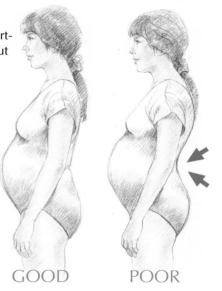

GOOD   POOR

Varicose veins
Varicose veins can appear in all three trimesters. Poor circulation due to standing or sitting for long periods of time can cause veins to swell and ache. When you are sitting, make gentle circles with your feet to increase circulation. Sit with your feet propped up on pillows several times a day. If you wear support stockings, put them on before getting out of bed in the morning.

A warning about saunas, hot tubs, and spas
You may be tempted to ease sore muscles or an aching back by getting into a hot tub, spa, or sauna. However, the high temperature can raise your body temperature to over 101° F (38° C) and reduce the oxygen flow to your growing baby. A warm (not hot) shower or tub bath is fine.

Begin to prepare your body for birth

Practice squatting for birth

The squatting position for either labor or birth is used effectively in many cultures. Squatting uses gravity to bring your baby down through the pelvis. It allows pelvic joints to move and make more room for your baby. Practicing the squatting position during your third trimester will condition your muscles for birth and help you to recover more quickly afterward.

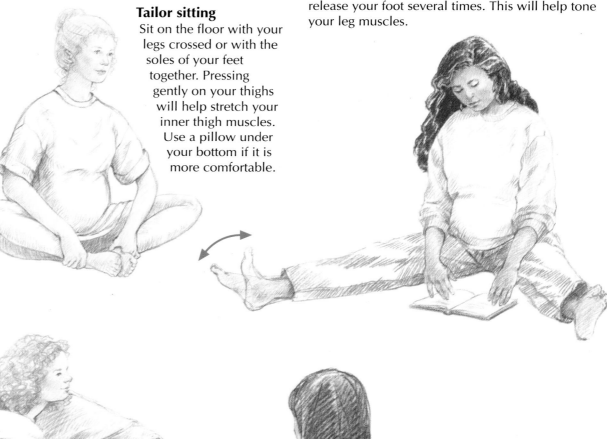

1. Spread your legs apart and keep your feet flat on the floor.
2. Slowly lower your weight onto your heels and toes.
3. Hold this position for 30 seconds or more.
4. Rise slowly. Don't bounce when you squat.

Here are two sitting positions that will help tone and gently stretch some of the muscles that you will use during birth.

Tailor sitting

Sit on the floor with your legs crossed or with the soles of your feet together. Pressing gently on your thighs will help stretch your inner thigh muscles. Use a pillow under your bottom if it is more comfortable.

You can use a partner for support either in front or in back of you.

Sitting with your legs apart

Sit on the floor with your back straight and your legs spread comfortably apart. Gently flex and release your foot several times. This will help tone your leg muscles.

43

Pelvic floor muscles

Your pelvis has a sling-like set of muscles that will stretch and make way for your baby at birth. You can learn to relax them effectively during birth if you do this gentle exercise. Imagine that you are stopping the flow of urine. Pull in and tighten the muscles around your vagina and anus. Hold your muscles in this position for as long as you can without strain. Relax them slowly. Repeat the exercise 15–20 times a day. Continuing pelvic floor exercises after birth will help these muscles regain their tone more quickly.

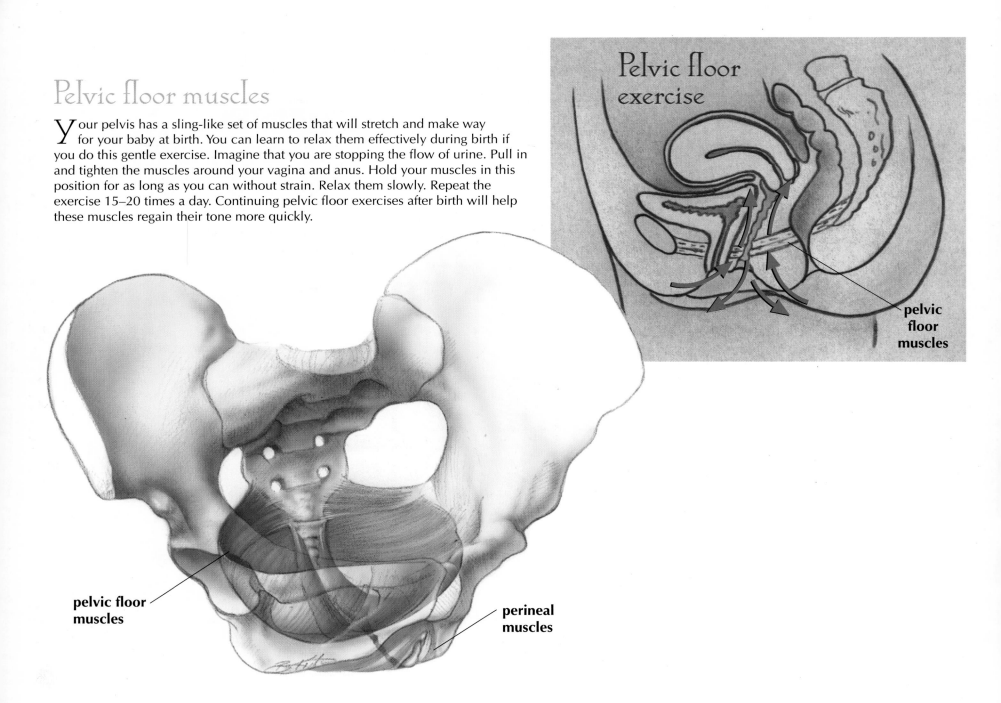

Pelvic floor exercise

pelvic floor muscles

pelvic floor muscles

perineal muscles

Timeline of pregnancy

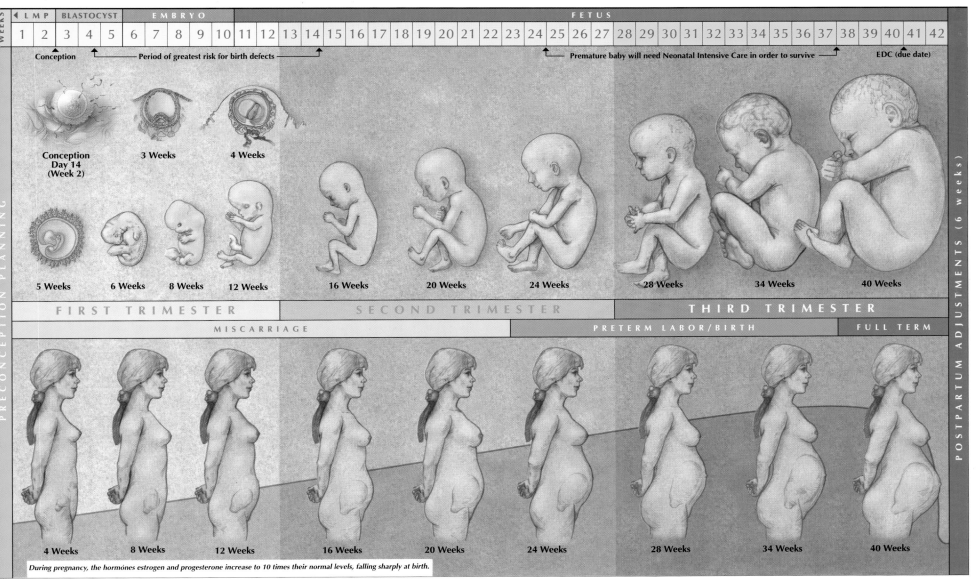

WEEKS	◀ L M P		BLASTOCYST			E M B R Y O																	F E T U S																				
	1	2	3	4	5	6	7	8	9	10	11	12	13	14	15	16	17	18	19	20	21	22	23	24	25	26	27	28	29	30	31	32	33	34	35	36	37	38	39	40	41	42

Conception — ◀ Period of greatest risk for birth defects ▶ — Premature baby will need Neonatal Intensive Care in order to survive — EDC (due date)

PRECONCEPTION PLANNING

POSTPARTUM ADJUSTMENTS (6 weeks)

Conception Day 14 (Week 2) — **3 Weeks** — **4 Weeks**

5 Weeks — **6 Weeks** — **8 Weeks** — **12 Weeks** — **16 Weeks** — **20 Weeks** — **24 Weeks** — **28 Weeks** — **34 Weeks** — **40 Weeks**

FIRST TRIMESTER — **SECOND TRIMESTER** — **THIRD TRIMESTER**

MISCARRIAGE — **PRETERM LABOR/BIRTH** — **FULL TERM**

4 Weeks — **8 Weeks** — **12 Weeks** — **16 Weeks** — **20 Weeks** — **24 Weeks** — **28 Weeks** — **34 Weeks** — **40 Weeks**

During pregnancy, the hormones estrogen and progesterone increase to 10 times their normal levels, falling sharply at birth.

The best place for your baby to grow is inside you. Every day—every week counts.

1 Month   2 Months   3 Months

4 WEEKS   **8 WEEKS**   **12 WEEKS**

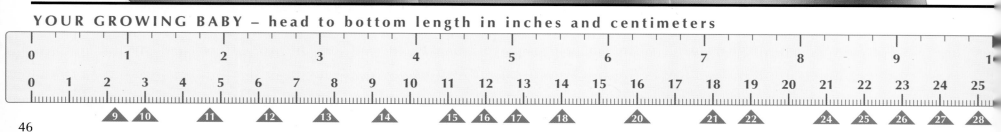

YOUR GROWING BABY – head to bottom length in inches and centimeters

| 0 | 1 | 2 | 3 | 4 | 5 | 6 | 7 | 8 | 9 | 1 |

| 0 | 1 | 2 | 3 | 4 | 5 | 6 | 7 | 8 | 9 | 10 | 11 | 12 | 13 | 14 | 15 | 16 | 17 | 18 | 19 | 20 | 21 | 22 | 23 | 24 | 25 |

9 10 11 12 13 14 15 16 17 18 20 21 22 24 25 26 27 28

46

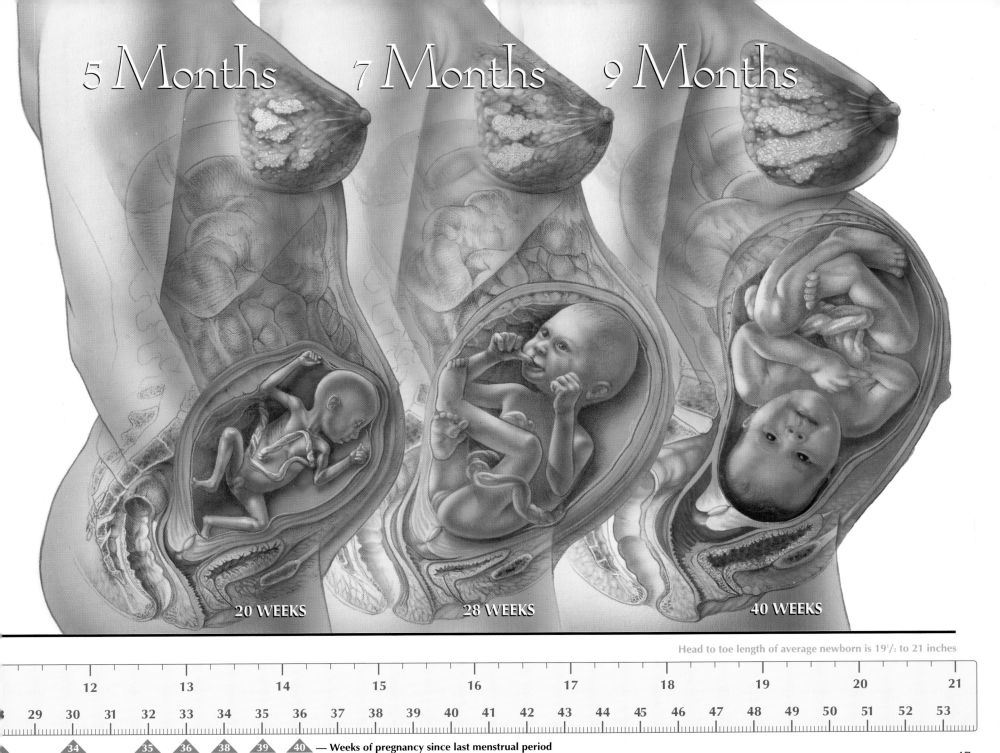

5 Months

7 Months

9 Months

20 WEEKS

28 WEEKS

40 WEEKS

Head to toe length of average newborn is 19¹/₂ to 21 inches

12   13   14   15   16   17   18   19   20   21

29 30 31 32 33 34 35 36 37 38 39 40 41 42 43 44 45 46 47 48 49 50 51 52 53

34   35 36 38 39 40 — **Weeks of pregnancy since last menstrual period**

Fetal development

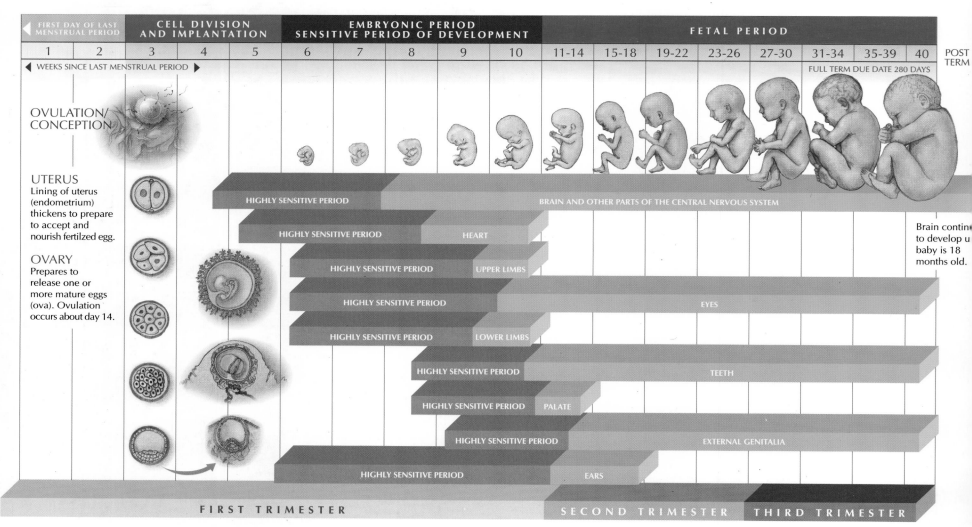

FIRST DAY OF LAST MENSTRUAL PERIOD	CELL DIVISION AND IMPLANTATION		EMBRYONIC PERIOD SENSITIVE PERIOD OF DEVELOPMENT					FETAL PERIOD									
1	2	3	4	5	6	7	8	9	10	11-14	15-18	19-22	23-26	27-30	31-34	35-39	40	POST TERM

◄ WEEKS SINCE LAST MENSTRUAL PERIOD ►

FULL TERM DUE DATE 280 DAYS

OVULATION/ CONCEPTION

UTERUS
Lining of uterus (endometrium) thickens to prepare to accept and nourish fertilzed egg.

OVARY
Prepares to release one or more mature eggs (ova). Ovulation occurs about day 14.

HIGHLY SENSITIVE PERIOD — BRAIN AND OTHER PARTS OF THE CENTRAL NERVOUS SYSTEM

Brain continues to develop until baby is 18 months old.

HIGHLY SENSITIVE PERIOD — HEART

HIGHLY SENSITIVE PERIOD — UPPER LIMBS

HIGHLY SENSITIVE PERIOD — EYES

HIGHLY SENSITIVE PERIOD — LOWER LIMBS

HIGHLY SENSITIVE PERIOD — TEETH

HIGHLY SENSITIVE PERIOD — PALATE

HIGHLY SENSITIVE PERIOD — EXTERNAL GENITALIA

HIGHLY SENSITIVE PERIOD — EARS

FIRST TRIMESTER   **SECOND TRIMESTER**   **THIRD TRIMESTER**

Protect your growing baby.
See your caregiver as soon as you know you are pregnant.
Go to <u>all</u> your prenatal visits.

1	ONE
2	
3	
4	
5	TWO
6	
7	
8	
9	THREE
10	
11	
12	
13	FOUR
14	
15	
16	
17	FIVE
18	
19	
20	
21	SIX
22	
23	
24	
25	SEVEN
26	
27	
28	
29	
30	EIGHT
31	
32	
33	
34	
35	NINE
36	
37	
38	
39	
40	
41	TEN
42	

FIRST TRIMESTER · SECOND TRIMESTER · THIRD TRIMESTER

Weeks — Months are shown in 28-day "lunar" months

7-8 Months

The developing pregnancy

Fetus

- There is less amniotic fluid and less room for your baby in your uterus now.
- Your baby's lungs, digestive system, and heat control system are still not mature. Your uterus is still the best place for the baby to grow.
- Weight at seven months: 2–3½ pounds
- Weight at eight months: 4–6½ pounds

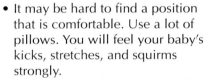

actual size

Fetal hand at 28-29 weeks

Father

- You may notice children more often in restaurants, parks, etc.
- Pregnancy is so intense at times that you may find yourself feeling tied down and wondering how you will feel after your baby is born.
- You may begin to feel protective toward the mother and your family.
- Continue to go to prenatal visits and birth education classes with the mother.

Mother

- You may feel heartburn and some indigestion due to the pressure on your stomach. Eating smaller, more frequent meals may help.
- Your belly is large and heavy. Your navel may become flat or it may even pop forward. You may feel that your body is being taken over.
- It may be hard to find a position that is comfortable. Use a lot of pillows. You will feel your baby's kicks, stretches, and squirms strongly.
- Your ankles and feet may swell.

Uterus

- The uterus grows from about three finger widths above the navel to just under the ribs. It pushes all the organs up, causing pressure on the lungs and stomach and sometimes pain in the rib cage.
- The top of the uterus tightens and releases. The uterus is getting ready for birth with these "practice" contractions. Usually, they are not painful.
  Call your caregiver if you are in doubt about what you are feeling.

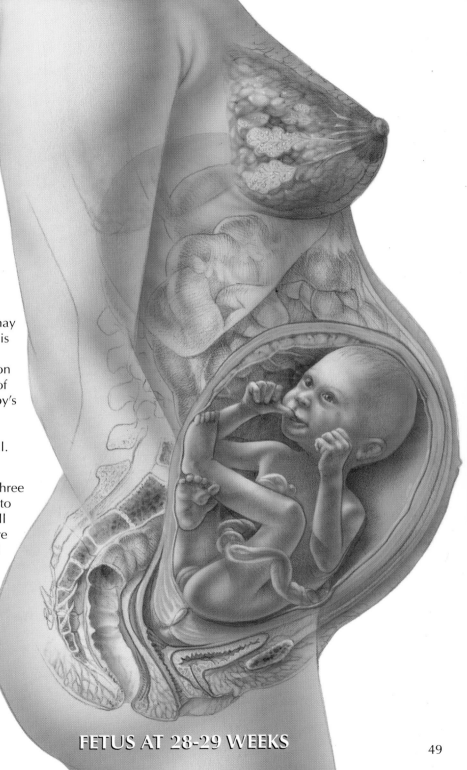

FETUS AT 28-29 WEEKS

49

Taking care of yourself

Taking time to eat well, exercise, and reduce stress is more important during pregnancy than at any other time in your life. Your baby depends on you.

Create a special time for yourself every day

Finding a peaceful place to relax, listen to music, and get in tune with your body helps you focus on keeping the demands of your life in balance. Use this time to write in your journal.

Touch relaxation

Learning to recognize tension in your body and how to release it from a specific part of your body helps to prepare for labor. Focus on releasing tension through your partner's hands as he touches and massages specific areas.

Visualization

When you are in a relaxed state, imagine your baby on its journey and visualize your body releasing your baby gently. Practice creating these images now and use them in labor.

How to avoid straining your back

Picking up objects from the floor

1. Squat down near the object, bending your knees.
2. Keep your back straight.
3. Pick up the object and hold it close to your body.
4. Push up using your leg muscles.

Getting up from a chair

1. Place one foot in front of the other.
2. Lean forward and put your hands on your knees.
3. Keep your neck and back straight.
4. Push off with your feet.

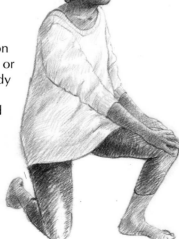

Avoid heavy lifting

1. Don't bend over at your waist to pick up anything.
2. Let children crawl into your lap rather than lift them.
3. Get help lifting heavy things up to or off of a high shelf.

The best way to take care of your growing baby is to take care of yourself.

Getting up from the floor

1. Roll to one side.
2. Bend your knees and hips.
3. Use your arms to push yourself up to your knees.
4. Place one foot flat on the floor.

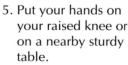

5. Put your hands on your raised knee or on a nearby sturdy table.
6. Use your leg and arm muscles to stand up.

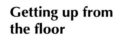

Making love during pregnancy

Ask your caregiver if there are any reasons to restrict your lovemaking during pregnancy. Usually, sexual intercourse is fine and can't harm your baby or cause infection. Here are a few guidelines:

• Gentle, tender sex is preferable to athletic sex.
• Choose a position that keeps the partner's weight off of the mother's belly and breasts.
• Be understanding and patient with each other.
• Soft caress and sensual massage with scented oils can be an enjoyable addition or alternative to intercourse.

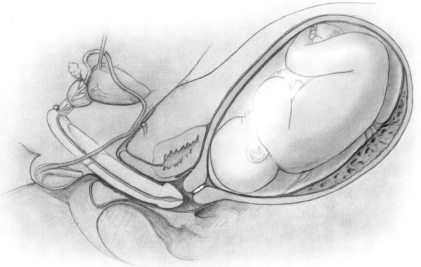

Getting to know your baby

Your baby can hear you

During your quiet time each day, talk and sing to your unborn baby. A baby's ability to hear is well-developed before birth. An unborn baby can distinguish between types of sounds, loud and soft sounds, and even different pitches of sounds. At birth babies seem to prefer higher pitched voices. Your baby has been hearing your voice all during pregnancy. If your baby is very active inside you at one period of the day, turn on soothing music. Sit down and rock in a rocking chair for 15 minutes or so and see if this calms your baby. The same music and motion may calm your baby after birth as well.

Your baby can feel your touch

You already know the sensation of your baby's kicks and turns inside you. Some babies move softly while others seem to be playing football inside you. Their personalities are developing even before they are born. *Gently* feel your baby's shape inside you. A long smooth area is likely to be its back. Lumpy areas are your baby's arms and legs. A firm, round area is the head. Sometimes you will see a small bump on your belly. It is likely that this is your baby's hand, foot, or elbow. If you gently massage the bump, the baby may pull its hand or foot back. Encourage your partner or children to share the experience of gently feeling your baby move inside you.

Establishing a new relationship with your parents

Within every family, family members have many different expectations of each other. You may be worried about how you will deal with your parents or your partner's parents and their expectations about how you will raise your child. Now is a good time to find out just what those expectations really are. You will need some help with managing daily life for a few weeks after your baby arrives. Who will help you? You and your partner need to define what kind of support you do and do not want from your families. After you have talked it over, you can talk with each of your families and do your best to be clear about what will be most helpful to you.

> "Pregnancy is a time for intensive building and rebuilding for families."
> — **Kitty Ernst, C.N.M.**

Learning about birth

Childbirth preparation classes

It is not uncommon for expectant mothers to feel fearful about giving birth. In birth education classes, you will learn about the process of giving birth, how to work with your labor, and what it feels like. Many classes offer practice in relaxation and breathing techniques that will help you cope with pain. Your partner will learn what to expect and what he can do to support you during labor. Some classes offer information or resources to help you learn how to care for your newborn and how to breastfeed. Here is a brief overview of the special focus of several different approaches to birth:

- **Eclectic:** Incorporates elements of various methods and techniques into comprehensive birth preparation.
- **Dick-Read:** Focuses on breaking cycles of fear, tension, and pain through knowledge, relaxation, and breathing techniques.
- **Lamaze:** Teaches specific techniques for breathing, relaxation, and labor support, as well as comprehensive birth education.
- **Bradley:** Emphasizes relaxation, slow abdominal breathing, and partner support.
- **Active birth:** Includes techniques of hatha yoga and actively changing labor and birth positions.
- **Odent:** Provides a quiet, gentle birth in a darkened room to welcome newborn.
- **Kitzinger:** Encourages the mother to be an active participant in birth rather than a passive patient. Emphasizes that birth is a natural, private, emotional, and psychosexual event.
- **Cesarean and VBAC:** Specialize in preparing parents for a cesarean delivery of their baby or in preparing for a vaginal birth after a cesarean delivery of a previous pregnancy.
- **Breastfeeding preparation:** Focuses on skills for breastfeeding.

Ask your caregiver for more information on these and other preparation classes offered in your community.

Finding a qualified instructor

Finding classes for a specific method of birth is less important than the quality of teaching and the teacher's relationship with the students. Effective classes will give you a sense of the rhythms and phases of labor and birth. The quality, philosophy, and format of classes can vary widely. While some classes are free, others are covered by insurance or have a separate fee. Smaller classes will make it easier for you to have your questions answered than large lecture-type sessions. Here are some questions to ask when you call to find out about different classes in your community:

- Who sponsors the classes?
- What is the training, certification, and affiliation of the instructor?
- Is child care provided for siblings?
- How many classes are there and how long is each session?
- Where are the classes taught?
- Is public transportation available to the class location?
- What is the class size?
- Is there a fee?
- Is there time for discussion and questions or is it lecture only?
- What topics are covered?
- What is the philosophy toward pregnancy and birth?
- What method is taught?
- Is there time to practice relaxation and breathing techniques in class?
- How much will you need to practice at home?
- How does the instructor use visual aids, models, videos?
- Can the instructor give references?

9 Months

FIRST TRIMESTER	1
	2
	3
ONE	4
	5
	6
TWO	7
	8
	9
THREE	10
	11
	12
SECOND TRIMESTER	13
	14
FOUR	15
	16
	17
FIVE	18
	19
	20
	21
SIX	22
	23
	24
	25
SEVEN	26
	27
	28
THIRD TRIMESTER	29
EIGHT	30
	31
	32
	33
NINE	34
	35
	36
	37
TEN	38
	39
	40
POST TERM	41
	42
	Weeks

Months are shown in 28 day "lunar" months

The developing pregnancy

Fetus

- Your baby's sucking reflexes are mature.
- The lungs and breathing reflexes are also mature.
- Your baby has lost most of the lanugo hair and some of the vernix that coated the skin.
- Your baby may settle into a quieter period for the last part of pregnancy.
- Weight at nine months: 7–7½ pounds

Father

- The pregnancy may begin to seem long and even endless for both parents at this point.
- Helping with groceries, cooking, and laundry makes a lot of difference during the last month. The demands of late pregnancy on the mother's body are heavy. She may be tired; hormone changes can make her forgetful.
- Set up the baby's crib.
- Learn the route to the birth center or hospital by the middle of the ninth month.
- Make sure your partner can reach you at all times.

Mother

- Your breasts produce more colostrum.
- The connecting tissues in your pelvis relax to make room for your baby's passage.
- You may need to urinate often because the baby is sitting on your bladder.
- Backaches can be severe, as the whole weight of the uterus and baby are tugging on your lower back.
- Difficulty sleeping and strange dreams about the baby or about birth are common.
- You may get a "nesting" urge and want to clean and organize everything. Rest instead.

Uterus

- The uterus is right up under the ribs and pushes on the lungs. This can cause shortness of breath and more heartburn.
- The uterine muscle is stretched very thin at the top. It begins to soften in the lower segment and lets the baby drop into the pelvis. This puts pressure on the cervix.
- More "practice" contractions may occur.
- The placenta is becoming less efficient.
- There is less amniotic fluid.
- Hormone levels start to change. They will fall sharply right after birth.

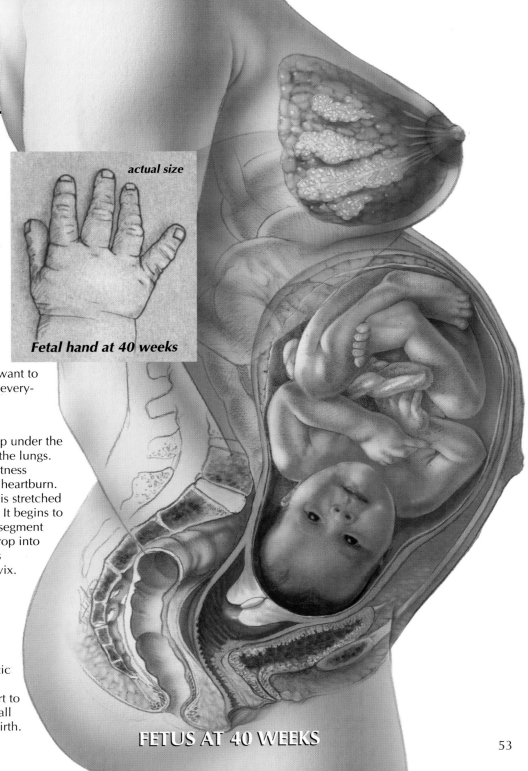

actual size

Fetal hand at 40 weeks

FETUS AT 40 WEEKS

Getting ready to give birth

You are seeing your caregiver every week now. You are being checked for signs of labor.

Check to see that:
- Your birth plan is written and a copy is in your caregiver's file. Take a copy in your bag.
- Your bags are packed. Your labor kit is ready.
- You know the route to the birth center or hospital, and the car has plenty of gas.
- You have your phone list, camera, and film.

When will your baby be born?

In late pregnancy your emotions range from serene contentment and excitement to anxiety and even outright impatience for your baby's birth. Remembering that your due date is an estimate and not a promise can be difficult. In uncomplicated pregnancies, almost 85 percent of all babies are born within a two-week window around the due date, with most of them arriving within the week after their due date. Only 5 percent are born on their due date.

"We are born with our very cells knowing how to give birth. We have only to learn to trust our bodies to do the work of labor."
—Harriette Hartigan

How will you know if you are in labor?

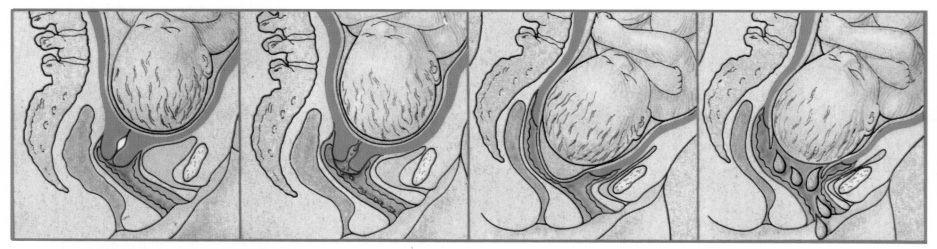

Early labor ripening and softening

Your cervix has stayed firm and closed during pregnancy to protect your baby. Hormones now cause it to soften like a piece of ripened fruit so that it is ready for labor.

Mucous plug and bloody show

A thick plug of mucus in the cervical canal begins to come out. Tiny blood vessels in the cervix bleed and cause "bloody show" from your vagina.

Effacement and dilatation

The cervix must get shorter and thinner (effacement) before it can open around your baby's head (dilatation). It may start to do this before labor begins.

Membrane rupture

Your membrane may break with a gush of almost two pints of fluid or with just a slow steady trickle of fluid. Membranes break during labor for about 88 percent of women.

How to time contractions

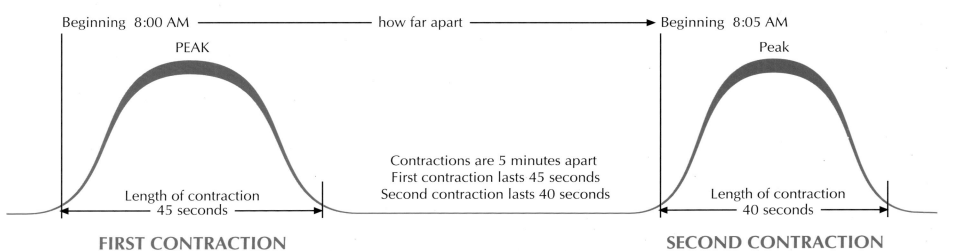

Beginning 8:00 AM ——————— how far apart ————————▶ Beginning 8:05 AM

PEAK

Peak

Contractions are 5 minutes apart
First contraction lasts 45 seconds
Second contraction lasts 40 seconds

Length of contraction
45 seconds

Length of contraction
40 seconds

FIRST CONTRACTION

SECOND CONTRACTION

TRUE LABOR	FALSE LABOR
CONTRACTIONS	
May be irregular at first. Usually become regular, longer, closer together, and stronger.	Usually irregular and short. Do not get closer together. Do not get stronger.
Walking makes them stronger.	Walking does not make them stronger.
Lying down does not make them go away.	Lying down may make them go away.
Usually felt in the lower back and radiate to the front.	Usually felt in the upper uterus and groin.
CHANGES IN THE CERVIX	
Cervix softens, thins, and opens.	May soften but little thinning or opening.
FETUS	
Begins to move into pelvis.	No significant change in position.

Pelvic station

Caregivers refer to the location of your baby within your pelvis as pelvic station. Before labor you may hear your caregiver say that your baby's head is still "floating" above your pelvis. When your baby's head is well into your pelvis, it is called "engaged" or at "zero station."

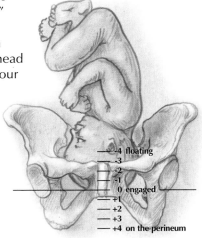

-4 floating
-3
-2
-1
0 engaged
+1
+2
+3
+4 on the perineum

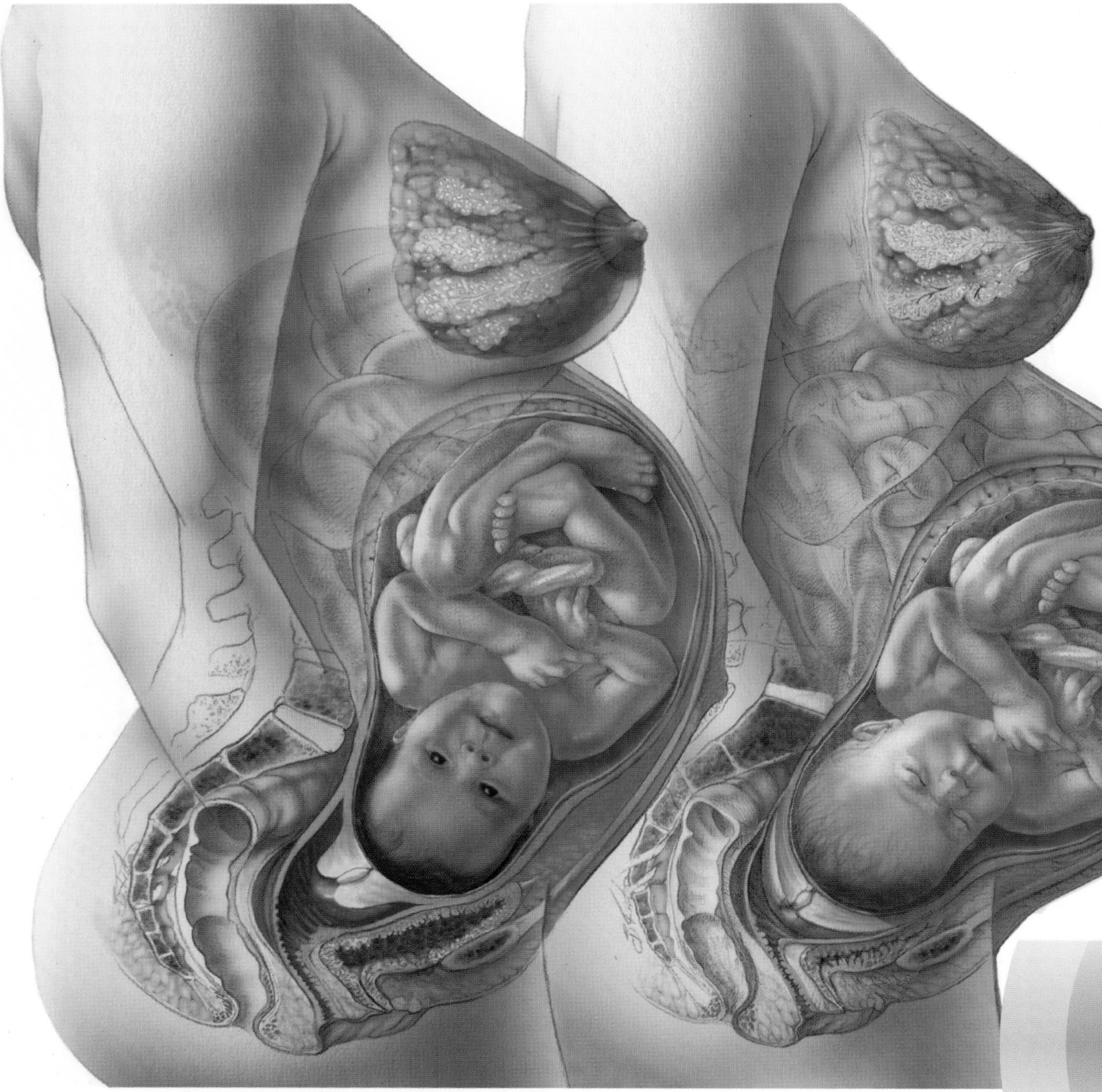

Lightening

After about 35 weeks, your baby fills all the space in your uterus. Most babies usually settle into a head-down position and seem to be resting for the coming labor and birth. If this is your first pregnancy, the baby moves down into your pelvis up to two weeks before labor begins. This is called lightening. If this happens, you will notice increased pressure on your bladder and pelvic floor muscles, but you will also be able to breathe a little better and have less heartburn.

How wide does your cervix need to open?

In late pregnancy, your cervix is as firm as the end of your nose. When it is fully dilated at the end of labor it is as soft as your cheek and almost as thin as paper. The dilatation of the cervix from 7–10 cm is called transition and is the hardest part of labor. It is also the shortest part of most labors. The tired mother needs loving support during this stage.

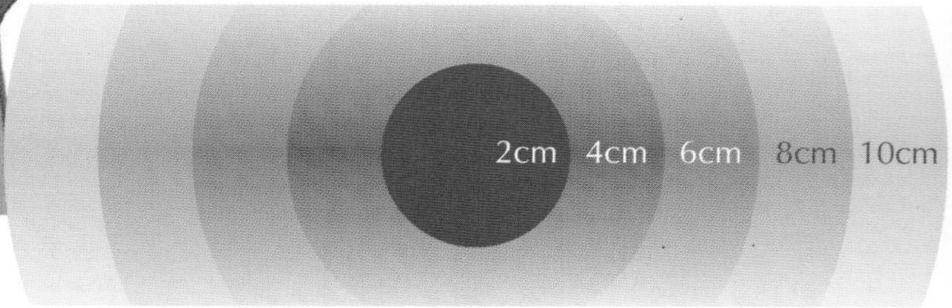

BEFORE LIGHTENING

AFTER LIGHTENING

2cm 4cm 6cm 8cm 10cm

Accurate centimeters of cervical dilatation

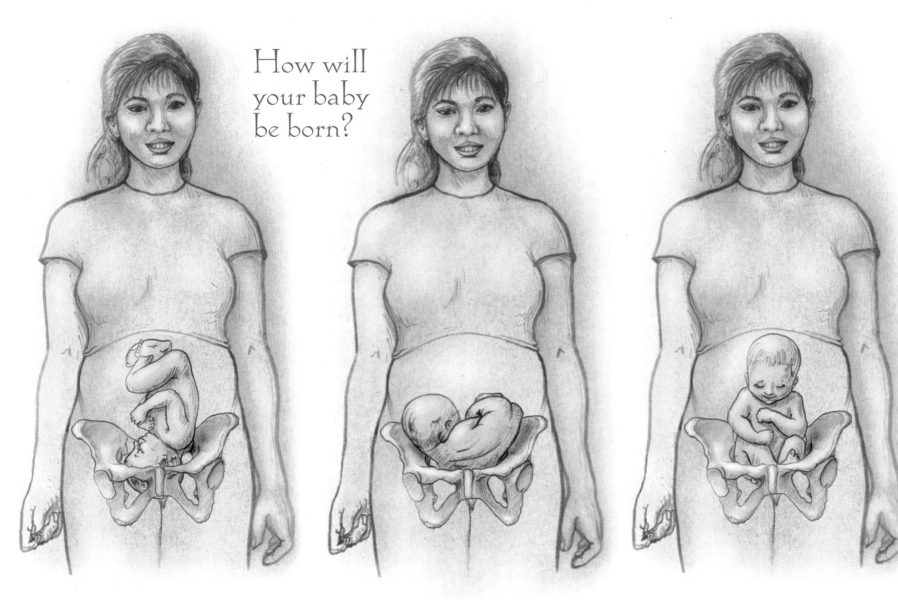

How will your baby be born?

HEAD FIRST (vertex)

Almost 95 percent of all babies are born head first. More than 80 percent of these babies are born vaginally.

SHOULDER OR ARM FIRST (transverse)

Only 1 percent of all babies are born shoulder or arm first. Almost all of them will be born by cesarean section.

BOTTOM FIRST (breech)

About four percent of all babies are born bottom first. Some of them will be born vaginally and some by cesarean section.

Types of Breech

COMPLETE

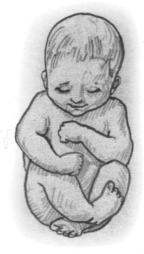

FRANK

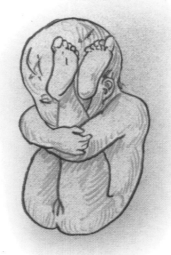

KNEELING

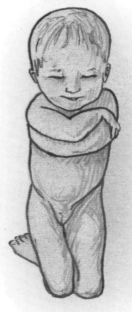

FOOTLING OR INCOMPLETE

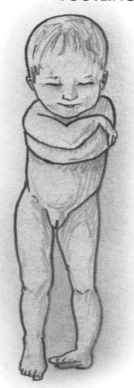 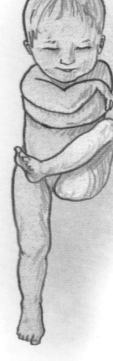

Surprise birth

Things you need to know:

STAY CALM—most fast deliveries are uncomplicated. Call 911 and ask for help and an ambulance.

1. Wash your hands with hot soapy water if possible.
2. Do not pull on the baby.
3. Tell the mom to pant and not push.
4. Let the head come out slowly. It will come out and turn to the side, then the shoulders will be born.
5. The baby will be slippery. Grip the baby under the arms. Put the baby on the mother's chest.
6. Do not pull on the cord.
7. Do not cut the cord.
8. Keep the baby and mother warm.

Birth procedures if there is time:

1. Get the mother in a semi-sitting position on a bed or on the floor.
2. Tell her to start panting to keep from pushing. Comfort and reassure her.
3. Put clean sheets or towels under her hips.
4. Cup one hand over the baby's head as it comes out. Apply light pressure to the head so that it does not pop out suddenly.
5. Let the baby's head turn to the side.
6. If the umbilical cord is looped around the baby's neck, gently slide it forward over the head.
7. Let the mother push down gently to deliver the shoulders. Let the baby slide out onto the bed.
8. The rest of the body will follow quickly once the shoulders are out.
9. Hold the baby with its head lower than its body for a few moments.
10. Dry the baby with a towel and put it on the mother's chest. Skin-to-skin contact is best.
11. Cover both of them with a blanket or coat.
12. Encourage the mom to breastfeed to control bleeding—even if she plans to bottle feed.
13. Wipe any mucus from the baby's nose.

14. Let the placenta come out on its own. Do not pull it out. Do not cut the cord.
15. Keep the placenta until help arrives—a medical professional should examine the placenta to be sure that all of it has been delivered.
16. Don't give the mother any medication.
17. Massage her abdomen lightly every few minutes.
18. Congratulate yourselves—you are a family.

Planning ahead for the weeks after birth

You are going to need help

Some family-oriented companies allow a new father to take paternity leave. This time can be an ideal way to get a family off to a good start. There is no doubt that a new mother will need help in doing daily tasks such as cooking and laundry. Friends and relatives can help clean, bring in meals, take care of older siblings, shop for groceries, etc. Caring for a newborn demands a great deal of time and energy of both parents. Plan ahead now, and get extra quantities of basic food and home supply items at the grocery store. Freeze some ready-to-cook meals. Accept offers of help after your baby arrives.

Make arrangements for your older children

Set up car pools to nursery school, day care, or school events that will happen in the first few weeks after your baby is born. Look ahead to birthday celebrations coming up and buy and wrap birthday presents to store away for future use. Some parents like to get a small present that the baby can give to the older siblings at birth or in the days after. Set up a special place, a chair or pile of pillows in your home, where you and the older child can read a book together and have quiet time while someone else cares for the baby.

Preparing to breastfeed

Find a lactation consultant before your baby arrives

In recent years a new and helpful professional has emerged—the lactation consultant. To get your breastfeeding experience off to a good start, contact a lactation consultant who can teach you breastfeeding techniques before your baby arrives. We no longer live in large extended families where breastfeeding information was easily shared. Lactation consultants are expertly trained to help new mothers get started breastfeeding and solve problems as they arise. A board certified lactation consultant will have the initials IBCLC after her name. Some consultants offer breastfeeding aids and breast pump rental stations as part of their practice. Lactation consultants usually offer classes and one-to-one teaching sessions. They will counsel you by phone, have you come to their office, or come directly to your home for instruction. Ask your caregiver or call a local breastfeeding support group for recommendations.

Find a pediatrician or family physician who supports breastfeeding

Pediatricians and family physicians have different philosophies of care just as obstetric caregivers do. Not all physicians are fully knowledgeable about breastfeeding techniques. Finding one who supports breastfeeding is important. Your lactation consultant may be able to suggest several names of pediatricians who support breastfeeding in your area.

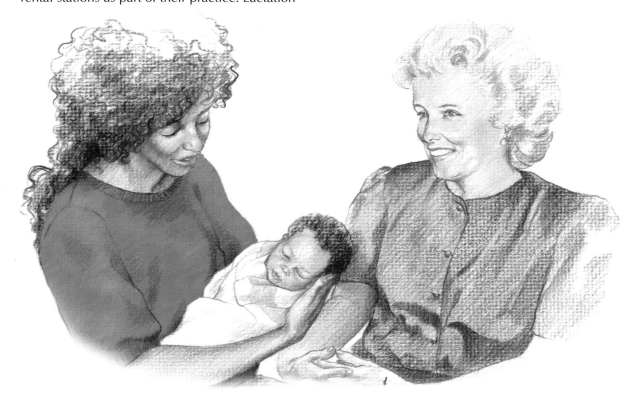

Questions to ask a pediatrician or family physician who will provide well child care for your baby:

- How many mothers in your practice breastfeed their infants?
- How many continue to breastfeed six weeks after their baby is born?
- How long do you recommend that a mother breastfeed her baby? (The American Academy of Pediatrics currently recommends breastfeeding for one year or longer.)
- Do you routinely recommend supplementing the diet of a breastfed baby with water or formula?
- If I have concerns or problems while I am breastfeeding will you refer me to a board certified lactation consultant or a breastfeeding counselor?
- How do you feel about mothers who return to work outside of the home and continue to breastfeed?
- When do you recommend introducing solids or vitamins to a breastfed baby?
- Do you have reference materials available in your office so that I may look up information about the safety of any drugs and medications that I may need to take while breastfeeding?

Set up a "breastfeeding station"

Find a room or place in your home where you feel comfortable and relaxed. Set up a "breastfeeding station" there. At least once a day, take the telephone off the hook while you feed your baby. Gather the following things for your comfort and convenience:

- A comfortable chair and a footstool
- Two or three pillows to use for support
- A small table next to the chair where you can keep a glass of water, juice, or milk to drink while you feed

- A small basket to keep a "burping" cloth, a change of diapers and clean clothes for your baby
- A small radio so that you can listen to your favorite music

Buy three good quality cotton maternity/ nursing bras

Maternity stores and departments carry specially designed bras which give firm support and have flaps which can be pulled down for easy feeding. Try them on before buying and be sure you can unhook and hook the flap with one hand. You will need three because your milk may tend to leak in the early days and you will want to wear a clean and dry bra. You may also want to get a supply of breast pads. Do not

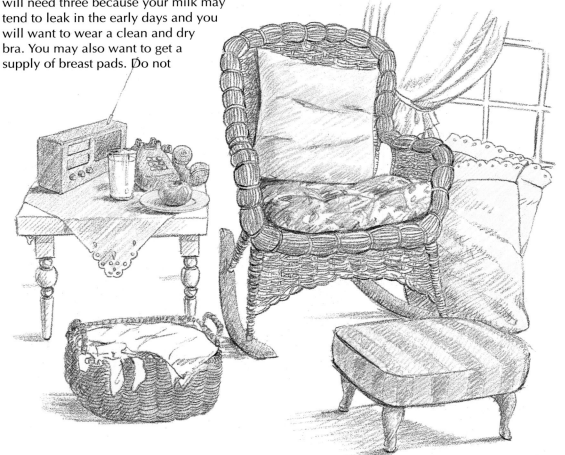

buy the kind with plastic liners, as they can hold moisture to your skin and cause problems. Breast shells are available that help collect any leaking milk and also help circulate air to sore nipples.

Breastfeed as soon after birth as possible

Breastfeeding in the first hour after birth is ideal if your baby is interested in feeding at this time. Breastfeed every two to three hours both night and day for the first few days to help bring in your milk supply.

Giving birth

The work of labor

We are used to being in control of our bodies. We decide when and where to walk, sit, stand, and use our muscles. One of the surprises of labor is the realization that your body begins to contract your uterine and abdominal muscles without your control or desire for this to happen. Contractions come and go like waves on a shore.

Your task in labor is to learn to cooperate with this rhythm and to let your body do what it knows how to do. Resisting labor with tension and anxiety can actually make it last longer. Cooperating with your contractions, relaxing, and trusting your body to do the work of labor are essential.

The uterus at full-term

Uterine muscle and ligaments
Uterus: At the end of pregnancy (full-term), the uterus is the largest muscle in the human body. Its unique structure lets it do the work of labor and then return to its normal size, ready for another pregnancy.
Ligaments: Thin round ligaments on the front of your uterus can over-stretch in late pregnancy when you cough, sneeze, or reach up. If this happens, you will feel a sudden sharp pain as the ligaments contract. Sit down until the pain is gone.

Abdominal muscles
The vertical bands of abdominal muscles may actually separate down the midline of your body in late pregnancy. If this happens, ask your caregiver or a physical therapist to show you exercises that will help knit the muscles back together after birth.

Pelvic floor and perineal muscles
The triangular arrangement of your pelvic floor muscles helps your baby turn correctly within your pelvis during labor and birth, following the line of least resistance.

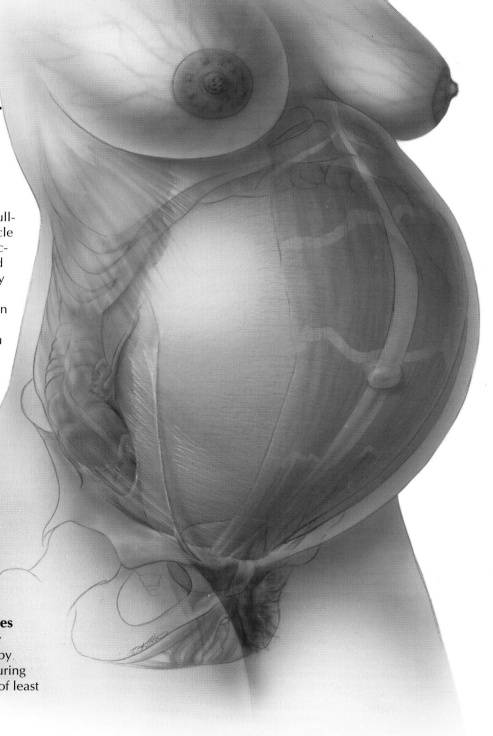

Coping with pain in labor and birth

Causes of labor pain

Labor pain is far different than pain caused by injury. It is not constant but comes and goes with each contraction of the uterus. Pain results from the thinning and stretching of the cervix as it opens around the baby's head and from the sensations of the birth canal stretching to open.

Dealing with the father's pain

The pain that an expectant father may feel during labor is emotional, but it is no less real than the mother's pain. We feel empathy for anyone we love experiencing pain. We would do almost anything to take it away. It is not uncommon for the father to blame himself for the mother's labor pain. Accept this feeling as normal and know that just being there with her is the greatest thing you can do to relieve her pain—no one else can give her such loving care and support.

Coping skills

Education: Learning about the natural process of giving birth and the choices you have for birth helps prepare both you and your partner.

Loving support: Having someone stay with you throughout labor and birth is perhaps the single most important factor in coping with pain and letting your labor progress.

Movement: No single position is comfortable throughout labor. Walking, squatting, or gently rocking your hips back and forth will help you be more comfortable. Change positions often.

Water: Taking a warm bath or shower to relieve aching muscles is a good remedy for pain at any time, including labor.

Relaxation: Tension release skills will help you relax and work with labor contractions and possibly shorten your labor.

Labor aids: Hot or cold compresses, soothing massage, and gentle pressure applied to any area that hurts can relieve pain.

Breathing: Consciously hearing your breath or doing patterned breathing will ensure the oxygen supply needed in labor.

Visualization: Creating positive mental images such as wellness and a peaceful, welcoming environment for your baby takes practice but can help to relax and to relieve pain.

Pain Medications

Following is a list of a variety of pain medications that are used during labor and birth. Consult with your healthcare provider about the possible benefits and risks of each.

Systemic Medications: Systemic medications include sedatives, tranquilizers, and narcotics, most often injected into a vein or into your IV. They are used to help you relax and induce sleep in early labor.

Analgesics: Analgesic medications are used during active labor to help dull labor pain. They can be injected into a vein or a muscle. Like systemic medications, they are primarily used in early labor to help you rest and conserve your energy.

Local Anesthesia: Local anesthetic medications are injected by a healthcare provider to numb a particular area during or after delivery (when stitches are needed); local anesthesia does not reduce labor pain.

Regional Anesthesia: Also called **epidural** or **spinal anesthesia**, regional anesthesia is used during birth to block pain in a wide region of the body while allowing you to remain awake. Medications are injected into the lower spinal area by an anesthesiologist. Regional anesthesia can also be used for a cesarean birth.

General Anesthesia: Used for birth emergencies, general anesthesia is given by an anesthesiologist. It causes total unconsciousness.

Note: Some women choose to utilize alternative treatments, such as hypnosis, acupressure, or acupuncture, instead of or in addition to traditional pain medications. If you are considering the use of an alternative method for coping with pain during labor and birth, consult with your caregiver about possible benefits and risks.

Coping with labor

Supporting a woman in labor

Labor support can be given by any compassionate or caring person who is willing to learn about the process of giving birth, understand its emotional and physical stresses, and learn how to relieve them. This person can be the baby's father or a friend or relative with whom the mother is comfortable. Some parents seek the services of a birthing assistant or doula to help them through labor in addition to having the father present.

The mother and support person need to become comfortable communicating about birth before it happens. Watching a movie of a birth together will be helpful, especially if the support person is not familiar with the normal sights and sounds of birth. Moans, sighs, and groans are all ways of relieving tension. Talk about what you saw and how you felt.

Guidelines for support:

- Create a quiet, soothing environment for labor with dim lighting and soft music.
- Observe her emotional state and respond to it calmly. She may welcome massage or back rubs one minute and then not want to be touched at all. This is normal.
- Don't expect her to respond to questions. She hears you but she may not be able to answer or talk much.
- Offer comfort and support, not criticism.
- Look for tension and use touch relaxation techniques to help her release it.
- Help her see pain as positive and productive. Her baby will be born soon.
- Breathe with her through the strong contractions of late labor.
- Provide distraction by helping her focus on an internal, visualized image or on a picture on the wall during contractions.
- Do not leave her alone.

Support during early to late labor

- Encourage her to eat lightly and sleep in early labor. She will need all the energy she can get.
- Time her contractions; write down how long they last and how much time passes between the start of one to the start of the next.
- Suggest that she change positions often. Upright or squatting positions are best for most of labor.
- Support her in your arms during a contraction.
- Massage her shoulders and back or apply pressure where her back hurts between contractions.
- A warm shower or bath provides a soothing break in a long labor and can help labor progress.
- Encourage her to urinate every hour.
- Give constant encouragement in short, positive statements: "That was a great contraction," "You are doing fine," or "You are making progress."
- Don't take any irritable comments she may make personally. The last part of labor is intense and short comments may be all she can manage.

Support during pushing and birth

- The contractions may subside briefly after she is fully dilated and before she starts to push. It may seem that labor has slowed, but this time allows her to rest before the great effort of pushing the baby out.
- Help her into delivery positions and support her as she pushes. Remind her that each push brings the baby nearer.
- Wipe her face with a cool cloth and then help her relax completely between contractions.
- When the baby's head is visible, encourage her to reach down and feel it. After the baby is born, stand by quietly for the next few minutes while the caregiver gives instructions.
- Giving birth is a massive life event. Be prepared for any reaction—from stunned silence to shouts of joy.

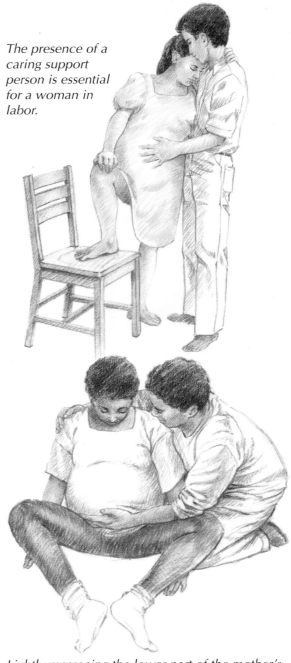

The presence of a caring support person is essential for a woman in labor.

Lightly massaging the lower part of the mother's belly in a back and forth motion can help to release tension.

Intervention and Technology

An intervention is a drug, device, or medical or surgical procedure used during labor or birth. Technology is the machinery or equipment used for intervention. Consult with your healthcare provider about the risks and benefits of each.

Intravenous fluids: Fluids given to help maintain your fluid level and blood pressure.

Amniotomy (artificial rupture of membranes): The amniotic sac is artificially ruptured, either to help start or speed labor or to use electronic fetal monitoring equipment.

Induction of labor: Amniotic membranes are loosened to help start labor; prostaglandin gel is placed in or near the cervix to help start labor; or a regulated amount of synthetic oxytocin is given in IV fluids to either start labor or to increase the intensity of contractions.

Fetal monitoring: There are several different types of fetal monitoring. A **fetoscope** is a stethoscope used to listen to the fetal heart rate; a **Doppler ultrasound** device can also be used to listen to the baby's heartbeat. **Electronic fetal monitoring** uses ultrasound to record fetal heart rate and contractions; it can be used intermittently or continuously during labor and birth. In **internal fetal monitoring**, an electrode is attached to the baby's head to record heart rate, and a pressure catheter monitors contractions. **Telemetry monitoring** uses radio waves to monitor fetal heart tones; it allows mobility because the device is attached to the mother's thigh.

Episiotomy: Incision to enlarge the vaginal opening just before birth.

Vacuum extraction: Suction cup applied to baby's scalp and traction used to help bring the baby through the birth canal.

Forceps: Spoon-like instruments applied to each side of baby's head to help rotate head to better position or to bring the baby through the birth canal.

Cesarean section: Baby is delivered through an incision in the mother's abdomen and uterus.

Relief for back pain in labor

Backaches are common to most laboring women. As your baby moves down through your pelvis it must turn in order to be born. If your baby turns to face your front instead of your back, the pressure of its head against your sacrum may cause a severe backache. Coping skills can help to relieve a backache during labor.

- Change positions. Walk, lean over the back of a chair or the labor bed, get on all fours, or lie on your side. Choose the position that best suits you, but do not lie on your back.
- Gently rock your pelvis back and forth.
- Use ice packs, a hot water bottle wrapped in a towel, or a heating pad. Hold it to the area that aches.
- Counter pressure may feel good during contractions or between contractions. Ask your support person to:
  —Press the heel of his or her hand against your spine.
  —Apply firm pressure to both sides of your spine just above your buttocks.
  —Gently rub your sacrum and lower back, moving his or her thumbs in a circular motion.

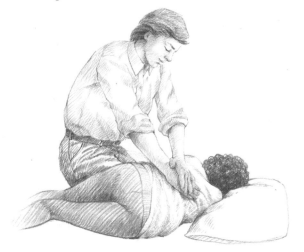

Relaxation

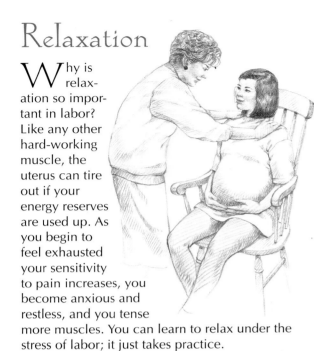

Why is relaxation so important in labor? Like any other hard-working muscle, the uterus can tire out if your energy reserves are used up. As you begin to feel exhausted your sensitivity to pain increases, you become anxious and restless, and you tense more muscles. You can learn to relax under the stress of labor; it just takes practice.

Touch relaxation

This method of relaxation teaches you to release tension to the warmth and touch of your partner's hand. Practice it with your partner daily for the last month of pregnancy and you should be able to relax under the stress of labor.

1. Mother lies or sits comfortably supported with pillows.
2. Mother tenses her shoulder muscles.
3. Partner gently puts his hands on mother's shoulders. Gentle, slow, light massage can be added to the touch.

4. Mother releases the tension in her shoulders and lets it flow out of her body toward the warmth of his hand.
5. Practice this tension–touch–massage–release exercise on other muscles. Areas that you tend to tense during labor are: face, head, and neck; shoulders, arms, and hands; small of your back and buttocks; legs and feet.

Breathing for relaxation

Slow, deep breathing is relaxing. Imagine that your contractions are like waves and that you are breathing slowly and deeply over the crest of a wave.

Positions for labor and birth

Upright positions

Moving and changing your position often helps your baby move through your pelvis and helps you to be more comfortable. Upright positions increase the effectiveness of your contractions and use gravity to help the baby descend. Walk between your contractions and support yourself by leaning on a wall or against your partner.

Side-lying positions

If you want to rest in bed for a while, lie on your side rather than on your back to allow maximum oxygen

flow to your baby and uterus. Put a pillow between your legs or use the side rails or stirrups attachment to support the weight of your upper leg.

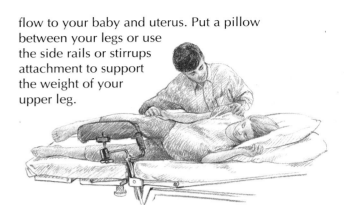

Kneeling positions

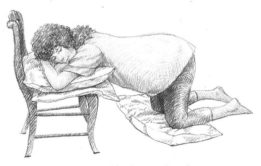

Getting on your hands and knees or kneeling at the side of the bed or against a chair helps take the weight of your uterus off of your back. Shifting positions helps make room for your baby to turn and move further into your pelvis.

Squatting positions

Squatting actually widens the dimensions of your pelvis as much as one centimeter and uses gravity to your advantage. Birthing beds often have a bar that can be attached to support you. You can squat and hold on to your partner's arm or the side of the bed. Or use a semi-standing position supported by your partner. Squat during the contraction and stand or sit between contractions.

Stages and phases of labor and birth

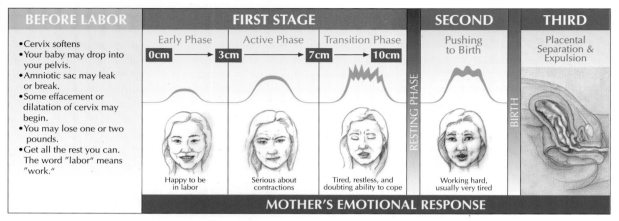

BEFORE LABOR	FIRST STAGE			SECOND	THIRD
	Early Phase	Active Phase	Transition Phase	Pushing to Birth	Placental Separation & Expulsion
• Cervix softens • Your baby may drop into your pelvis. • Amniotic sac may leak or break. • Some effacement or dilatation of cervix may begin. • You may lose one or two pounds. • Get all the rest you can. The word "labor" means "work."	0cm → 3cm	3cm → 7cm	7cm → 10cm		
	Happy to be in labor	Serious about contractions	Tired, restless, and doubting ability to cope	Working hard, usually very tired	

MOTHER'S EMOTIONAL RESPONSE

Internal exam during labor

Vaginal examination (internal exam) is done two or three times during labor. It can be done by your caregiver, a labor nurse, or physicians in training (interns or residents). It tells your caregiver:

• How much effacement (thinning and shortening of the cervical canal) has occurred
• How much dilatation has occurred
• How your baby is presenting (head first, feet first, etc.)
• What position your baby is in (facing your side, front or back)
• How far your baby has moved down into your pelvis

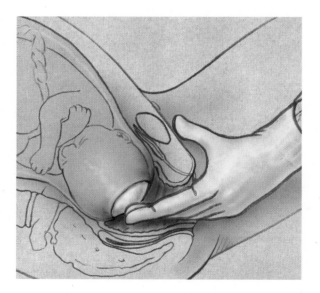

What makes labor start?

There is still no certain answer, but when labor starts appears to be controlled by a combination of hormone levels that are changing in the mother and hormones that the baby starts to produce when it is ready for birth. You may have heard that many babies are born at the time of a full moon. However, a recent study of 50 million births in the U.S. shows that the highest number of births occur 21 days into the lunar cycle—seven days after a full moon.

How long does labor last?

Labor and birth usually happen more quickly after your first baby. Here are some averages for first-time mothers. Keep in mind that wide ranges of time are still considered normal.

Early labor (1–3 cm) – eight hours
Active labor (3–7 cm) – five hours
Transition labor (7–10 cm) – 30–90 minutes
Pushing baby out – a few minutes to hours

Different labors

No two labors are exactly the same. Normal labors can be quick and intense or long. Most labors and births are uncomplicated. Cooperating with your body is an important part of letting your labor progress. Here are a few labor terms you may hear from caregivers or friends who have given birth:

• **Induced or intensified labors** are usually stimulated with drugs for medical reasons and require more use of technological intervention and monitoring.
• **Prodromal labor** has a long early phase before active labor takes over. Sometimes this can be due to the baby's size or position as it enters the mother's pelvis.
• **Posterior or "back labor"** is caused by the baby rotating to face the mother's front instead of her back as it moves through her pelvis. The pressure of the baby's head causes moderate to severe backache for the mother.

Progress in labor

Many factors influence how your labor and birth will progress. It is the unique combination of these factors that make the experience of labor and birth different for each woman.

- The size of your pelvis
- The size of your baby's head
- Presentation (head first or bottom first) of your baby as it enters your pelvis
- Position (facing your side, back, or front) of your baby as it enters and moves through your pelvis
- Descent (downward movement) of your baby into your pelvis
- Rotation (turning) of your baby through your pelvis
- The rate of effacement (thinning and shortening) and dilatation (opening) of your cervix around your baby's head or bottom
- The strength of the uterine contractions
- Your ability to relax
- Your coping techniques
- Your confidence level
- Your emotional state
- Your energy level
- The caring presence and support from your partner, a friend, a birth assistant, or a doula

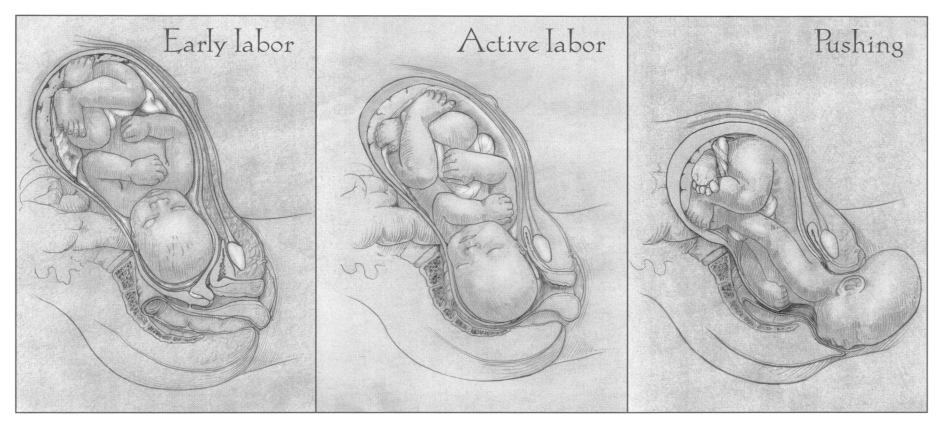

Early labor

Active labor

Pushing

Your baby faces your side as it enters your pelvis. During a contraction, the uterus becomes firm at the top while it relaxes and opens at the bottom.

The contractions open the cervix around your baby's head in the same way a turtleneck sweater stretches open as you pull it over your head.

By the time your cervix is fully open (dilated), your uterus has become a thick and powerful muscle at the top, ready to push your baby down the birth canal. Your baby needs to turn within your pelvis to face your back in order to be born.

Complications in labor and birth

In most cases, labor and birth is a healthy and uncomplicated process for both mother and baby. Occasionally, situations do arise that need active medical management to resolve. Sometimes cesarean section is the optimum choice for delivery.

Cesarean delivery

Cesarean section is the surgical delivery of the baby through an incision made in the mother's abdomen and uterus. It is usually the fastest route to deliver a baby when an obstetric emergency arises. It may also be scheduled (elective cesarean) for known medical conditions that affect the health of either the mother or the baby. Like any abdominal surgery, it carries a greater risk of infection and complication for the mother. It will also take her longer to recover after birth than a vaginal delivery.

Reasons for cesarean delivery:

• Unusual position of the baby
• The baby's head is too large or the mother's pelvis is too small
• Medical conditions in the mother such as hypertension or diabetes
• Distress in the baby during labor
• The umbilical cord drops down ahead of the baby and is compressed during labor contractions
• The placenta covers the opening of the uterus or it pulls away from the uterus during labor

Partners or support people may still share the birth experience in most cesarean deliveries. In fact, the partner has an important role in remembering everything he sees and recounting it to the mother later. Depending on the circumstances, cesarean section is done under regional anesthesia, which allows the mother to remain awake, or general anesthesia, which puts the mother to sleep during the birth.

Vaginal birth after cesarean (VBAC)

Depending on the reasons for the first cesarean, a mother may give birth vaginally without problems in other pregnancies that follow. Vaginal birth after cesarean is a healthy alternative for both mother and baby because it reduces the risks of complications associated with abdominal surgery (cesarean section).

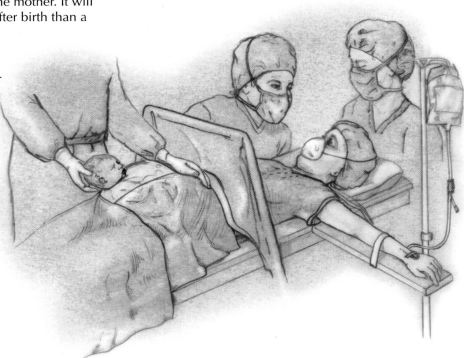

Newborn—the first days

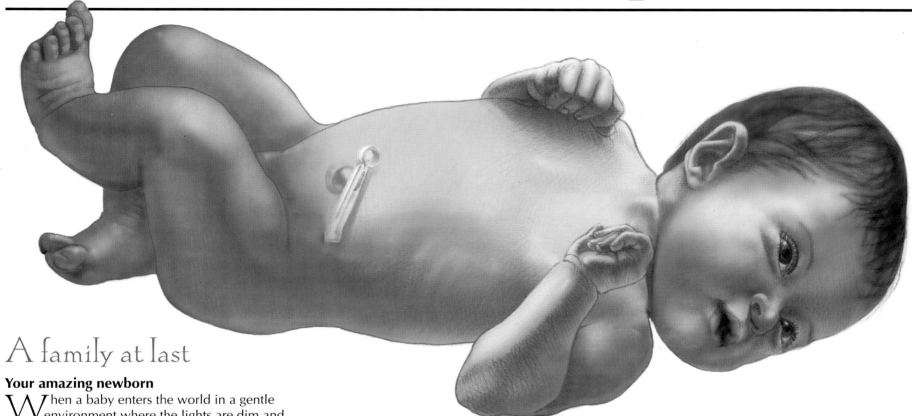

A family at last

Your amazing newborn

When a baby enters the world in a gentle environment where the lights are dim and the distractions in the room are minimal, it will open its eyes wide and gaze intently at its mother (and father) with a look that is both searching and yet unbelievably full of wisdom. When a baby is held skin-to-skin and is warmed by the mother or father, it becomes calm and wide awake. It seems to be taking in and trying to make sense of the new world.

This remarkable period can begin moments after birth and last for 40 minutes or so. After the first hour a newborn generally goes into a deep and contented sleep. Talk to your caregiver before birth about how you can create this kind of peaceful environment to welcome your baby to a new life. Until the moment of birth, you and your baby have journeyed as one, and the welcoming is the first chance you have to communicate your love as you become a family.

Studies show that all babies arrive with the ability to express a full range of emotions, from joy and fear to sadness and anger. Parents are often surprised to find that their baby can yawn, grimace, smile, and stare intently. The mother (or father) who has repeatedly sung lullabies to her baby before birth will be astonished to find that her newborn will recognize her voice, turn its head toward her, and be comforted by the familiar song.

The senses of touch, sight, hearing, taste, and smell do not suddenly start functioning at birth. They begin developing prenatally, as early as the first trimester, to prepare the baby to interact with its family and with life in the world outside the womb.

We once thought of newborns as little beings who had limited ability to interact with their environment. Now, we know that newborns enter our world with many abilities:

- Babies can see clearly at a distance of 8–10 inches. Interestingly, this is about the distance between the mother's face and the baby's face while breastfeeding.
- They can tell the difference between salty, sweet, bitter, or acidic tastes.
- They respond most to human voices and already know their mother's voice. They will respond and turn their heads to the source of sounds they hear. Newborns are able to block out sounds that bother them.
- They are sensitive to smell. Within six days, a breastfed baby will be able to identify its mother by sense of smell alone.
- Touch, closeness, and warmth are essential to a newborn's sense of security. Newborns use touch to contact, explore, and understand their new world. Studies have shown that when humans or other animals are deprived of physical contact, they do not learn to relate well to others of their species.

Newborns arrive with several interesting reflexes. Some will disappear within a few weeks or months and reappear later. For instance, a newborn whose head and weight are well supported can take steps, placing one foot in front of the other. A newborn may startle at loud noises, throwing his arms out and then pulling them back into his chest. If you press gently on a newborn's palm he will open his mouth. Newborns have abilities that we are only beginning to recognize and understand.

Family bonding

The sensory feeling of your newborn placed skin-to-skin on your chest or the father's chest is one that will long be remembered. Everything you imagined or wondered about your baby is suddenly real and in your arms. These first moments are not only to be savored, they can be the foundation of your sense that you and your baby belong to one another. Skin-to-skin contact with your baby, eye and voice contact, and the chance to explore with wonder the tiny, compact body of your newborn are all part of the bonding process. Ideally, this can begin within the first hour after birth in a dimly lit room where you are given a time of privacy as a new family.

Bonding is, however, a process and not a single moment. Some mothers need a few moments to rest and reorganize after the exhaustion of a hard labor. Others will reach down and help deliver their child right onto their abdomen. The father may want to cut the cord. Siblings may have attended the birth or may have been brought in by friends or grandparents right after birth to join the family celebration. All of these things are choices in normal birthing.

The sight of your newborn—its skin wrinkled and wet, perhaps still coated with some of the vernix, its head molded from the journey through the birth canal—can be quite a shock at first. You may even feel just a little squeamish about touching your baby. Yet for many parents the absolute wonder of the moment they view their baby blocks out everything and everyone else in the room.

The mother's condition right after birth

The moment of birth brings sudden and total relief from the sensations of pressure that you have been feeling as you work with strong pushing contractions. You are likely to experience an intense range of emotions—joy, relief, sadness, concern, etc. You may feel suddenly cold and start to shiver. This is a normal reaction of your body to the stress that it has been under. Your contractions stop as your baby is born. Within a few minutes you will feel another contraction starting. This last contraction forces the placenta to peel away from the wall of your uterus. The contraction will also push the placenta out of your body. The nursing staff will examine it carefully to see that no part of the placenta and amniotic sac is left inside you. A sample of blood will be taken from the cord so that they can determine your baby's blood type. If you have had an episiotomy (an incision made to enlarge the vaginal opening), it will be repaired after the placenta has been delivered.

Newborn appearance

Most parents have an image of what their newborn will look like at the moment of birth that is often quite different from reality. The "newborn" babies that you see in television shows are usually about four to six weeks old. Your newborn baby has just finished a long journey and like any traveler needs a little time to recover.

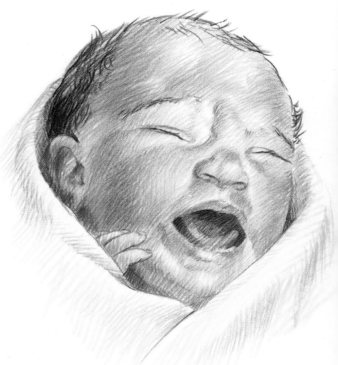

Vernix

Vernix caseosa is the white, creamy substance that serves as a protective skin covering for your baby while inside you. Most of the vernix will be gone by the time your baby is born, but some may still remain in folds and creases of the skin.

Skin color

Your baby's skin will flush with color as he takes his first breath. A newborn's hands and sometimes feet may be blue-gray because of slow blood circulation. African-American babies will be lighter in skin color for the first few days.

Molded head

Your newborn's head may be long and molded at the back from the pressure of the birth canal. Molding is temporary; the baby's head will return to normal a few days after birth.

Swollen scrotum

A male infant will often have swollen and sometimes reddened genitals at birth because of maternal hormones that have passed to him during pregnancy.

Vacuum extractor "cap" and forceps bruise

Skin bruises and swelling may result from the pressure of the vacuum suction cap or from forceps. The swelling will go down within 24–48 hours after birth. The baby's head may be tender for the first 24 hours or so.

Newborn procedures

Suctioning of baby's mouth and nasal passages

Upon birth, a bulb syringe is used to remove any mucus or amniotic fluid from your newborn's mouth and nose. This is done so that he will not inhale any fluid when he takes his first breath.

Clamping and cutting of the umbilical cord

The umbilical cord will be clamped in two places and cut within the first few minutes after your baby is born. Some fathers like to cut the cord. If your partner is interested in doing this, ask your nurse-midwife or physician how it can be arranged. The umbilical area should be kept clean and exposed to the air as much as possible to help the healing process. The cord stump will dry up and fall off within seven to 10 days after birth. Your baby needs to be sponge bathed until the cord stump is well healed.

Apgar assessment

Your caregivers will monitor your condition and your baby's condition. You may hear numbers assigned to your baby right after birth and again a few minutes later. This is an Apgar scoring system that checks your baby's heartbeat, breathing efforts, color, vigorous movements, and reflexes. It is a rapid method for caregivers to answer the question "Does this baby need help right now?"

Eye medication

State law requires treatment of newborns' eyes within one hour of birth with medication to prevent a serious eye infection caused by exposure to possible sexually transmitted disease in the mother's vaginal tract. Infected infants can suffer permanent blindness. Tetracycline or Erythromycin ointments are used as well as silver nitrate. Both ointments cause less irritation to the eyes than silver nitrate.

Vitamin K injection

Because newborns have low levels of vitamin K for the first few weeks, almost every newborn receives vitamin K shortly after they are born. An intramuscular injection of water-soluble Vitamin K is given to the baby to prevent excessive bleeding in the neonatal period when normal body production of the vitamin is low. This procedure is usually done in most newborn nurseries shortly after birth.

ID bands

If your baby is born in a hospital, identification bands are attached to the infant's ankle and wrist soon after birth. A band is also placed on the mother's wrist. The bands have identical identification numbers and last name.

Footprinting

Footprints are made of each newborn soon after birth and usually become part of the birth certificate along with the mother's fingerprint. If requested, the birth center or hospital staff will usually make an additional copy of the baby's footprints for the parents to keep.

Weighing and measuring

Your baby will be weighed and measured soon after birth. The average weight of a full-term infant is 3,500 grams (7½ lb). Ninety-five percent of infants weigh between 2,500 grams (5½ lb) and 4,259 grams (9½ lb). Infants usually experience some weight loss during the first three to five days of life, possibly as much as 10 percent of the infant's birth weight. This is usually regained in eight to 12 days. The average length of a full-term infant is 51 cm (20 inches). Ninety-five percent of infants will be between 45–56 cm (18–22 inches).

Pediatric exam

In addition to the Apgar assessment, newborns are usually examined by a pediatrician or by someone trained to do an immediate newborn evaluation. At the moment of birth a newborn's body must make rapid and significant changes in the functioning of many of its major organs. If the baby shows any signs of distress, immediate action can be taken.

Temperature control

A newborn is not able to regulate its body temperature very well and can become cool quickly. After birth, a small cap is placed on your baby's head right away. We can lose up to 40 percent of our body heat through our heads; the cap helps your baby stay warm. Putting your baby skin-to-skin with you is nature's best way of keeping your baby's temperature stable. A warmed blanket can be placed over both of you.

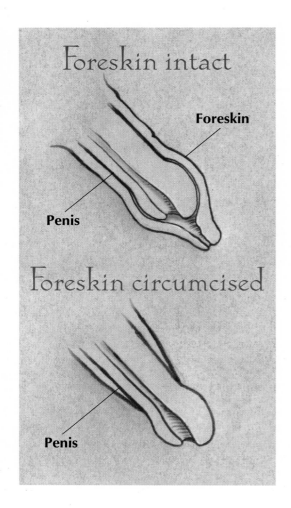

Foreskin intact

Foreskin

Penis

Foreskin circumcised

Penis

The circumcision decision

Circumcision is the surgical removal of the foreskin from the tip of the penis. The procedure is routinely done with a local anesthetic, as it may be painful. If you have a boy, you and your partner will need to choose whether or not you want to have him circumcised or leave his foreskin intact. The issue of circumcision continues to be controversial. For some, circumcision is a religious ritual; for others, it is a cultural preference. You and your partner should weigh the risks and benefits and discuss your beliefs about circumcision before your baby is born.

Parenting and breastfeeding

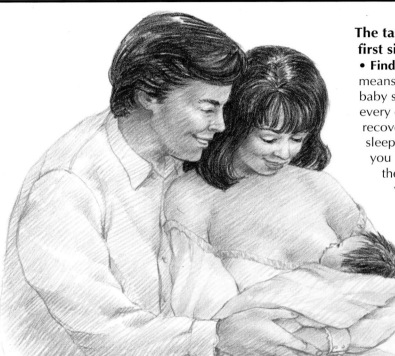

The challenge of becoming parents

Parenting is an extended learning experience—our children are our teachers. Family counselor Edward Deci remarks that "getting pregnant is easy, being pregnant is easy, and parenting is hard." Your first few weeks with a new baby can be difficult, especially if you are first-time parents. It is common to feel panic about not being able to handle this sudden 24-hours-a-day, 7-days-a-week job.

The tasks of parenting in the first six weeks

- **Finding some way to get rest:** This means lying down whenever your baby sleeps. Lack of sleep will make every other part of parenting and recovery harder to handle. It's a "skip sleep now and pay later" situation. If you do not take care of yourself in the first two weeks after birth, you will set your recovery back six to eight weeks. Your body needs rest in order to heal. Your baby needs you constantly. Fatigue is your single worst enemy in the first few weeks.

- **Getting through hormonal "crash":** Within hours after birth, your hormone levels drop. It will take about six weeks for your body to adjust. Meanwhile, you may experience mood swings—remember that this is natural.

- **Getting to know your baby:** Your baby may have a very different style and personality than the one you imagined in the child of your dreams. Spend time playing with your baby to learn how to balance your rhythms together.

- **Balancing visitors and your needs:** You are thrilled to show off the baby, but visitors can be wearing on your strength. Put a sign on the door announcing your baby's birth along with a note, "Mother and baby are resting." Add birthday information to any phone message recording.

- **Hearing "advice" and doing what you feel is right:** Even if you are new at parenting, no one knows your baby's needs better than you do. Believe in yourself and remember that your baby does not know that you aren't an old hand at this parenting business. If you are confused or worried about what you have heard, ask your caregiver, birth educator, or lactation consultant to clarify the information for you.

- **Finding time alone together with your partner:** This is something you will have to make happen now and in all your years of parenting to come. With everything that needs to be done for the baby and the family, even two of you are sometimes not enough to go around. When this happens you tend to neglect each other. Get a babysitter and spend time alone with your partner; you can discuss family plans and listen to each other's needs.

- **Accepting help:** Gladly accept any offers of help with meal preparation, housework, laundry, or shopping. If you are doing it all yourself, you won't be enjoying your little one.

- **Learning your baby's cries:** Crying is the only language your baby has. Babies have different cries when they are hungry, tired, bored, frightened, or when they just need to cuddle. Listen carefully and trust yourself. You know your baby.

- **Keeping things in perspective:** This Pie of Life shows how relatively short these "crowded times" really are in the larger view of your life. The newborn period is very memorable for its intensity, but it is truly a short time. None of the blessings or the difficulties of any phase of your baby's development will last. There is always something new to learn in the next phase. Be gentle and patient with yourself along the way.

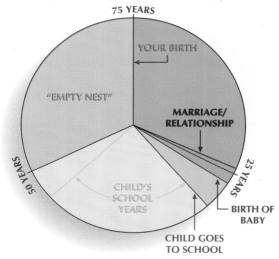

Keeping your baby safe from harm

Babies are born to explore their world and they become mobile quickly. One of your largest responsibilities will be to keep your baby safe. Here are some of the leading causes of injury and death to infants under one year of age and suggestions on how to prevent them:

Preventing crib accidents
Cribs can have unexpected dangers for a baby.
- Choose a crib that does not have decorative cutouts in the headboard or footboard. It is possible for a baby's head to become wedged into such places.

- Be sure slats on the crib are no more than 2³/₈ inches apart for the same reason. No slats should be broken or missing.
- Choose a firm mattress and don't use a pillow for your baby or leave one in the crib. A child can suffocate.
- Don't hang toys on a string or cord tied to the side or tied across the crib.
- Don't leave the side of the crib down even for a minute while your baby is in it.

Preventing burns
Hot liquids can scald and burn a small child.
- Use place mats instead of a table cloth. A baby can be burned by grabbing a table cloth and pulling a cup of hot coffee, tea, or soup over onto itself.
- Don't hold your baby while you are drinking any hot liquid.
- Run cold water in the faucet before you put your baby in the tub.
- Don't put your baby down or place a crib near a space heater. Blankets can fall on the heater and catch fire.
- Keep fire screens in front of all fireplaces.

Preventing falls and accidents
A fall or car accident can injure a baby's head and brain.
- Never leave your baby unattended on a sofa, chair, or changing table—even for a minute.
- Never put your baby down to sleep alone on an adult-size bed.
- Put a gate at the top and bottom of any stairs.
- Do not use a baby walker. The American Academy of Pediatrics recommends a ban on the sale of all walkers. Walkers roll down stairs easily and allow your baby to reach places that are not safe.
- Put your baby in a car seat for every ride. Put it in the center of the back seat, facing backward. Fasten the seat belt and harness tightly.

Preventing choking
Babies love to put everything they pick up into their mouths. They can choke on many small things around the house. Try to keep small objects out of their reach. Keep your baby in the same room with you and learn to react quickly to pull things out of its mouth. Here are just a few of the things that a baby might put into its mouth that can cause choking:
- Safety pins
- Beads
- Earrings
- Coins
- Paper clips
- Marbles
- Game parts
- Balloons
- Barrettes
- Nails
- Screws

Babies can also choke on foods such as:
- Hot dogs
- Grapes
- Nuts
- Popcorn
- Raisins
- Hard candy
- Marshmallows
- Pretzel sticks
- Raw carrots
- Chewing gum

Keep your purse and plastic bags out of your baby's reach.

Preventing poisoning
Many common household items can be hazardous to a small child.
- Keep all house plants off the floor and out of reach. Many of them are poisonous.
- Keep all medicines locked up.
- Keep cleaning products locked away: kitchen and bathroom cleaners, soaps and bleach.
- Keep lawn and garden products locked away: pesticides, plant sprays, fertilizers, car cleaners.

Preventing drowning
A baby can drown in as little as two inches of water.
- Never leave your baby alone in a bathtub.
- Keep diaper pails or buckets out of reach.
- Keep the toilet lid down.

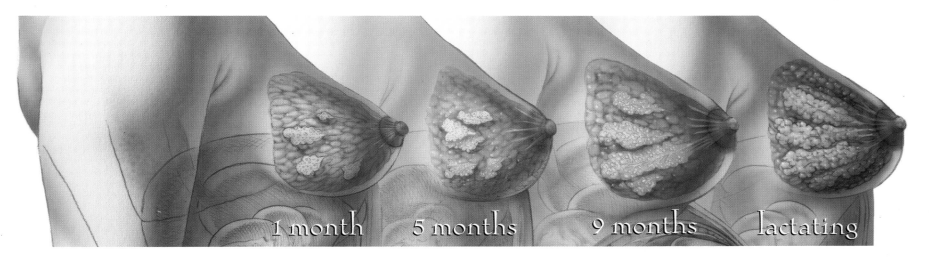

1 month   5 months   9 months   lactating

Sudden infant death syndrome

The American Academy of Pediatrics recommends that infants be placed on their backs for sleeping. There is a higher incidence of sudden infant death syndrome (SIDS) in infants who sleep on their stomachs or sides. There are a few situations in which placing infants on their stomachs may be preferred (i.e. reflux), but this decision should only be made with the input of a healthcare provider.

Breastfeeding your baby

Changes in your breasts

One of the first effects of hormones on your body during pregnancy is to prepare your breasts to be able to breastfeed your baby at birth. Although society and commercial advertising frequently tell us that breasts are valued for their sexual appeal, the true function of the human breast is to provide the best form of nutrition and disease protection for a newborn infant through the production of breastmilk.

At your baby's birth, your breasts are ready to supply nourishment. Your baby gets valuable immunization protection from your first milk (colostrum). Your breastmilk will come in about 24–48 hours after giving birth. Your breast tissue may contain extra fluid for a few days before your daily milk supply is established, and your breasts may be firm and swollen during this time. If you have chosen not to breastfeed, you will be given an injection at the time of birth to dry up your milk. You may feel some discomfort in your breasts for the first few days.

Benefits of breastfeeding
Benefits for you

• Breastfeeding helps you to get your figure back faster. Weight loss can be easier because of the extra calories that breastfeeding requires. Breastfeeding also helps your uterus return to normal size.
• Your breastmilk is always ready. No mixing, measuring, or heating. There is no need for sterilization or refrigeration, and there is nothing to clean-up.
• Nighttime feedings are easy. You can cuddle your baby in bed with you and still get your rest while she feeds.
• Breastfeeding saves you money.

- Going out is easier because breastfed babies are easy to take along. No equipment is needed.
- Breastfeeding is a warm and cozy time for both of you. It helps you feel close to your baby and feel confident about yourself as a mother.
- You can read stories to an older child while you breastfeed your baby. It's a great time for everyone to cuddle in bed together.

Benefits for your baby

- Breastmilk is the perfect food for your baby. Its nutritional content is just what your baby needs. Your breastmilk changes to meet your growing baby's needs. Breastmilk substitutes cannot do this.
- Your early breastmilk, called colostrum or "first milk," gives your baby protection against disease because immunities from your body pass to your baby.
- Breastmilk is gentle to your baby's stomach and easy to digest. He will have less colic, constipation, and diarrhea.
- A breastfed baby's bowel movements typically have less odor than those of a bottle-fed baby.
- Breastfed babies generally require fewer doctor visits and fewer trips to the hospital. They also have fewer earaches and colds than bottle-fed babies do. In addition, breastfed babies have fewer cases of asthma, food allergies, and eczema (skin conditions).
- Breastfeeding is special to your baby. At the same time you are feeding him, you are giving him the skin-to-skin contact that helps him feel comforted and secure. Breastfeeding stimulates all of his senses. He will love this special feeding time you have together.

> "Breastfeeding is the most precious gift a mother can give her baby. The most compelling reason is that human milk is specific for the growth and development of the human infant. It protects against infections, some chronic illnesses, and cultivates a special relationship between mother and infant."
>
> **Ruth A. Lawrence, M.D., pediatrician**

Positions for breastfeeding

Before you start a feeding, get into a comfortable position with your arms and back well supported by pillows. Put a pillow under your baby.

Getting started

- Support your breast with four fingers underneath your breast and your thumb on top.
- Bring your baby's nose up to the level of your nipple.
- Tickle your baby's lips with your nipple.
- Wait until her mouth opens wide.
- Pull your baby up and onto your breast.
- Be sure her lips are rolled outward and that her tongue is under your nipple.

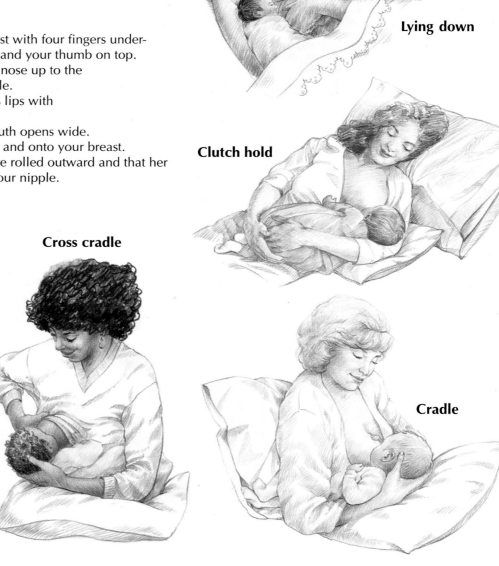

Lying down

Clutch hold

Cross cradle

Cradle

Postpartum

Changes in your uterus

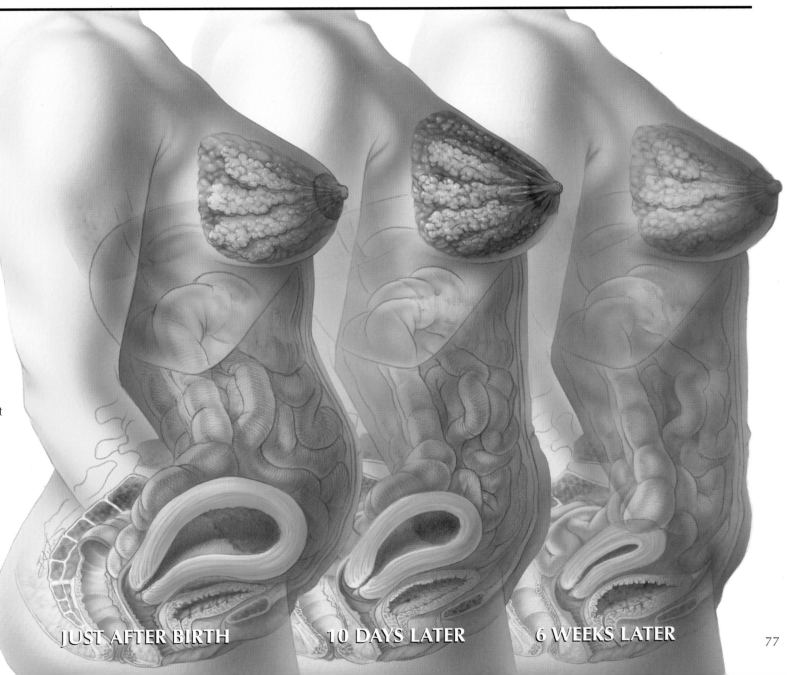

Your uterus will be about the size of a grapefruit after birth. It will stay contracted to keep from bleeding too heavily. Over the next six weeks, the uterus will return to its normal pear-like size. The place where the placenta was attached will heal completely, leaving no scar tissue. As the uterus heals, you will have a bloody discharge that is bright red in the beginning and then becomes pink, brownish, and finally almost a clear or yellowish fluid.

JUST AFTER BIRTH **10 DAYS LATER** **6 WEEKS LATER**

Adjusting to a child-centered lifestyle

Adjustments for the mother

Almost every new mother feels overwhelmed by the tasks that face her. Fatigue and hormonal changes contribute to this feeling of being unable to cope. As your body heals, you should begin to get over these bouts of postpartum sadness and feel better about your ability to cope. For some new mothers, however, clinical depression sets in, and they are unable to recover without help.

The signs of lasting depression that need professional treatment are:
- Extended feelings of hopelessness
- Guilt about not being the mother that you wanted to be
- Withdrawing from contact with others
- Sleeplessness in spite of exhaustion
- Lack of concentration
- Fears that you will harm the baby
- Feeling constantly "out of control" and unable to cope with daily living
- Not wanting to touch the baby
- Confusion and disorientation
- Unusual fears
- Eating disorders

If you experience any of these signs, seek help right away. Many caring professionals and support groups are available who will help you turn things around. There is no need to struggle alone and feel that no other mother has felt like this. Many new mothers have, and with help, they are fine today.

The needs of new mothers:
- Come to terms with their birth experience; it is a powerful event in any woman's life
- Make some time for themselves
- Be mothered themselves so that they can feel secure in their new role
- Feel nurtured and protected
- Avoid isolation, and talk with other mothers and friends
- Share the parenting role with their partner
- Talk openly about their feelings
- Rest, exercise, and eat healthy foods
- Take a break from the mothering role and go out with her partner and friends
- Don't worry about housekeeping tasks for a few weeks; accept offers of help from family and friends

Postpartum warning signs

Call your caregiver right away to report any of the symptoms listed below. They may indicate infection that needs to be treated with prescription drugs.
- Fever
- Increasing pain from episiotomy
- Burning when you urinate
- A painful, red area on your breast
- A return to bright red bleeding from your vagina after it had been brown or pink
- Foul odor from your vaginal discharge
- Slight opening of a cesarean incision
- Swollen, painful red area on your leg that is hot to the touch

Getting back in shape

Start slowly and don't overdo it. Here are a few exercises that you can begin to do each day. Always check with your caregiver first. Repeat each one five times to start and increase to 10 times each. Stop if you feel any pain or have any bleeding.

1. **Head to chest:** Lying on the floor with your knees drawn up comfortably, lift your chin to your chest. Hold for a moment, and then lower your head.
2. **Pelvic tilt:** Lying on the floor with both knees drawn up, gently rock your pelvis, pressing it into the floor, and then release.
3. **Pelvic floor:** Slowly contract the muscles that surround the vagina and hold for a count of three, and then release slowly.
4. **Leg slides:** Lie on the floor with one knee bent to a comfortable position. Slide your leg forward until your foot reaches the ankle on your extended leg. Pull your knee back up slowly. Repeat with the other leg.
5. **Foot flexes:** Alternate pointing your toes and flexing your foot.

At your postpartum checkup, your caregiver may suggest that you join an exercise program for new mothers. Check with your birth center, hospital, community center, or health club to see if it offers exercise classes especially for women who have just given birth. You can also rent or buy videos and books on pregnancy and postpartum exercise.

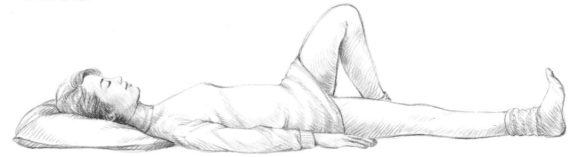

Adjustments for the father

The shock of the day-and-night needs of the new family keeps many new fathers off balance for a while. Your delight with the baby isn't lessened by her needs, but the exhaustion factor of interrupted sleep for everyone can be difficult when you have to put in a full work day the next morning. You realize that your lifestyle has indeed changed. There is little spontaneity in these first few weeks, and even the best-laid plans seem to go awry.

Some fathers experience conflicts. If they increase their work hours so the mother can stay home with the baby, they may be limiting their own time to interact with their newborn. Partners who used to share household tasks before birth can both feel unfairly burdened after the baby's arrival. There is simply too much for everyone to do. Agreeing ahead of time on who does what can help reduce tension.

If you and your partner discussed before birth how you want to raise your child, you will be better prepared to deal with problems than couples who suddenly realize that they have opposite opinions on how to raise their baby. The same holds true for agreeing on how to respond to unsolicited advice from family and friends.

As much as you may have looked forward to resuming a normal sex life, you may be surprised to find that the mother is totally absorbed in coping with the baby's needs and has little interest in sex for several weeks. Delaying intercourse for three to six weeks after the baby is born is common. The mother's tissues are sore and need time to heal for her to be comfortable.

"Before you were conceived I wanted you. Before you were born I loved you. Before you were here one hour I would die for you. This is the miracle of life."

— **Maureen Hawkins**
The Miracle

Resuming contraception

A woman who has given birth will ovulate *before* she has her first menstrual period again. Using contraception from the very first time you make love after the birth is important. Women have become pregnant again in the month immediately after giving birth because they failed to start using contraception again. Your body needs time to recover and heal from your pregnancy. Your hormones need to return to their normal level. Getting pregnant immediately after giving birth is not only too heavy a strain on your body, it is not ideal for anyone's needs—father, mother, baby, or siblings. Take care to plan ahead.

If you are breastfeeding, estrogen or progesterone contraceptive pills are not recommended, as some of the hormones will pass through your breastmilk to your baby.

Breastfeeding may also cause a further delay in the return of menstrual cycles. Don't wait to start using contraception—you don't know when menstruation will begin again, and you will ovulate before any signs of your period appear. Talk with your caregiver about the contraceptive choices available to you, and discuss your personal preferences with your partner.

Our children are our gifts to the future

If this is your first child, the first hours of life with your newborn will give you a profound appreciation for what it is to be totally responsible for another human life. At the moment of your baby's birth, you are transformed from being the receivers of care to being the providers of care. How will you survive? How will you know if you are being a "good" parent? Often, parenting is a matter of sorting out what is important. Here are seven ideas for constructive parenting:

1. **Believe in yourself.** If you thought people gave you unwanted advice when you were pregnant, you will be amazed at how many opinions there are about how you should raise your child. Parenting is a constant learning curve, and in a sense, you will always be a first-time parent to your oldest child. There will always be a first time you are dealing with a two year old, a 10 year old, a teenager, or a young adult. Trust yourself to be a caring parent. Even though you are learning, you still know your child better than anyone else.

2. **Meet your child's need when the need is there.** The intensity of the first weeks with your newborn won't last. Babies grow and change at an astounding rate, and so do their needs. Yet, today is the only thing that counts. Meeting your child's needs as they arise in the first few weeks and months will make him feel that the world is a safe and welcoming place. He will learn confidence and trust—in your love and in himself.

3. **Understand that even before birth your child has a specific personality.** Your job is to observe and discover that personality and to find out how you can help it blossom. Some parents waste months, even years, in an effort to mold a child into a personality that is against his or her basic nature. A shy, quiet child can be drawn out, but no amount of coaxing will ever turn him into an extrovert. The child who is a natural extrovert will seldom feel content sitting quietly and playing by herself. Learn, respect, and nurture the differences in each of your children.

4. **Think about what you say and do in front of your children.** How you approach problems in your own life can teach your child either adaptability or dependence. Rather than greet

each difficulty you face with dread and apprehension, show your child that new experiences and change can be fascinating. When your child wants to try something new, reacting openly and positively to his ideas teaches the beauty of possibilities and the acceptance of making mistakes. Saying "That will never work—you should do it this way" teaches fear of trying and lack of self-confidence. Read child development books on positive ways to discipline. Learn from other parents and professionals about constructive ways to talk to children.

5. **Teach your children a sense of wonder and appreciation for nature, art, music, and literature.** Take walks in the park and go to the zoo. Go to an art museum and take your child along in a back carrier so she can see the paintings too. Play different kinds of music every day or sing songs to your child. Borrow books from the library and read aloud to your child every day right from the start. Reading helps to develop her language skills and her love of learning. Show your child the variety that life offers.

6. **Welcome the idea that your child is also your teacher.** As adults we have layered our lives with complicated schedules and cluttered our thinking with many unnecessary rules and ideas. Children are so wonderfully straightforward. Take joy in their simple observations, and let them show you new ways to look at and experience life. Relax and be as spontaneous as they are. Your life will be richer for it.

7. **Every day of their lives, tell your children that you love them.** With all the tasks of daily care such as bathing, feeding, and transporting, it is easy to assume that your children know they are loved—after all, you are doing so many things for them. If you can do only one thing for your children every day, let each of them know that he or she is loved. Tell them again and again. Love is truly the only thing that matters. A child who knows that he is loved will feel secure and learn to give love to others as he grows up. A child who knows that she is loved will have the emotional foundation that will help her to accomplish any goal she sets in life. What better future can we give our children? What better gift can we give them than love?

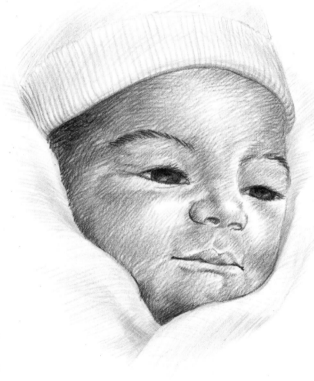

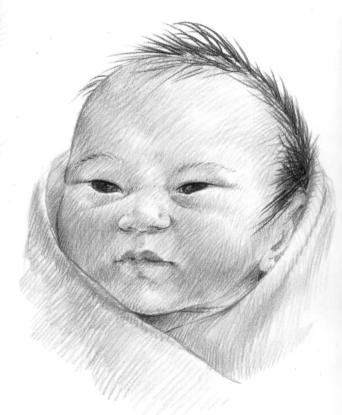

Reading and video resources for childbearing

Many of the books and videos listed in this section are available through Childbirth Graphics. Call 1-800-299-3366, ext. 287, to place your order.

Before you conceive

Preconception planning

Books

Rothman, Barbara Katz, et al. **The Encyclopedia of Childbearing**. New York: Henry Holt and Company, Inc., 1993.

Sussman, John R., M.D., and Levitt, B. Blake. **Before You Conceive, The Complete Prepregnancy Guide**. New York: Bantam Books, 1989.

Visscher, Harrison C., M.D., F.A.C.O.G., et al. **Planning for Pregnancy, Birth, and Beyond**. New York: The Penguin Group, 1990.

Infertility

Books

Harkness, Carla. **The Infertility Book**. Berkeley, CA: Celestial Arts, 1987.

Shapiro, Constance Hoenk. **Infertility and Pregnancy Loss**. San Francisco, CA: Jossey-Bass Publishers, 1988.

Choosing a caregiver

Books

Jacobs, Sandra and the American College of Nurse-Midwives. **Having Your Baby With a Nurse-Midwife**. New York: Hyperion, 1993.

Poole, Catherine M. and Parr, Elizabeth A., C.N.M. **Choosing a Nurse-Midwife**. New York: John Wiley and Sons, Inc, 1994.

Fetal development and pregnancy

Fetal development

Books

Bolane, Jamie Eloise, **Life Unto Life**. Waco, TX: WRS Group, Inc., 1988.

Flanagan, Geraldine Lux. **The First Nine Months of Life**. New York: Simon and Schuster, Inc., 1962.

Nilsson, Lennart and Hamberger, Lars. **A Child Is Born**. New York: Delacorte Press/Seymor Lawrence, 1990.

Videos

The Miracle of Life, Nova/Sweriges Television, 1986.

Knowing the Unborn, Pre Birth Parenting, 1987.

Pregnancy – general

Books

Carter, John Mack, et al. **The Good Housekeeping Illustrated Book of Pregnancy and Baby Care**. New York: Hearst Books, 1990.

Curtis, Glade B., M.D., F.A.C.O.G. **Your Pregnancy Week by Week**. Tucson, AZ: Fisher Books, 1989.

Eisenber, Arlene, Murkoff, Heidi E. and Hathaway, Sandee E. **What to Expect When You're Expecting**. New York: Workman Publishing, 1991.

Johnson, Robert V., M.D., et al. **Mayo Clinic Complete Book of Pregnancy and Baby's First Year**. New York: William Morrow and Co., Inc., 1994.

Kitzinger, Sheila and Bailey, Vicky. **Pregnancy: Day by Day**. New York: Alfred A. Knopf, Inc., 1994.

Kitzinger, Sheila. **The Complete Book of Pregnancy and Childbirth**. New York: Alfred A. Knopf, Inc., 1993.

Lansky, Vicki, et al. **Complete Pregnancy and Baby Book**. Lincolnwood, IL: Publications International, Ltd., 1993.

Rugh, Roberts, Ph.D., Shettles, Landrum B. Ph.D., M.D. **From Conception to Birth**. New York: Harper & Row, 1971.

Samuels, Mike, M.D., and Samuels, Nancy. **The Well Pregnancy Book**. New York: Fireside, 1986.

Simkin, Penny, R.P.T., Whalley, Janet, R.N., B.S.N. and Keppler, Ann, R.N., M.N. **Pregnancy, Childbirth, and the Newborn**. New York: Meadowbrook Press, 1991.

Stoppard, Miriam, M.D. **Conception, Pregnancy and Birth**. New York: Dorling Kindersley, 1993.

Stukane, Eileen. **The Dream Worlds of Pregnancy**. Barrytown, NY: Station Hill Press, Inc.,1985.

Van Der Meer, Antonia. **Great Expectations**. New York: Dell Publishing, 1993.

Visscher, Harrison C., M.D., F.A.C.O.G., et al. **Planning for Pregnancy, Birth, and Beyond**. New York: The Penguin Group, 1990.

Noble, Elizabeth. **Having Twins**. Boston: Houghton Mifflin Company, 1991.

Videos

Pregnancy, Mom, and the Unborn Baby, Human Care, 1990.

From Conception to Birth, LifeCircle, 1992.

Teen pregnancy & parenting

Books

Brinkley, Ginny, Sampson, Sherry, and Cooper, Gail Sprat. **You & Your New Baby.** Atlantic Beach, FL: Pink, Inc!, 1991.

Lindsey, Jeanne Warren. **Teens Parenting: Discipline from Birth to Three**. Buena Park, CA:

Morning Glory Press, 1991.

Barr, Linda, M.A. and Monserrat, Catherine, Ph.D. *Teen Pregnancy, a New Beginning.* Albuquerque, NM: New Futures, Inc., 1992.

Videos
Just a Beginning – Prenatal Care for Teens, Television Network, 1988.

Morning sickness

Books
Erick, Miriam, R.D., M.S. *No More Morning Sickness.* New York: The Penguin Group, 1993.

Video
Morning Sickness: All Day and All Night, Lemon-Aid Films, Inc., 1992.

Emotional journey

Books
Gardner, Joy. *Healing Yourself During Pregnancy.* Freedom, CA: The Crossing Press, 1987.

Peterson, Gayle, Ph.D. *An Easier Childbirth.* Berkeley, CA: Shadow and Light Publications, 1993.

Massage in pregnancy
Stillerman, Elaine, L.M.T. *Mother Massage.* New York: Dell Publishing, 1992.

Fathers and pregnancy

Books
Marshall, Connie, R.N. *The Expectant Father.* Citrus Heights, CA: Conmar Publishing, Inc., 1992.

Shapiro, Jerrold Lee, Ph.D. *When Men Are Pregnant.* New York: Dell Publishing, 1987.

Shapiro, Jerrold Lee, Ph.D. *The Measure of a Man, Becoming the Father You Wish Your Father Had Been.* New York: Perigee, 1995.

Nutrition and exercise

Books
Worthington, Bonnie and Williams, Sue Rodwell. *Nutrition in Pregnancy and Lactation.* St. Louis, MO: Mosby, 1988.

Exercise

Videos
Pregnant and Fit, Fit Video, 1987.

Everymom's Prenatal Exercise and Relaxation, Everymom's and Crystal Vision, 1989.

Problems in pregnancy
HIV/AIDS in pregnancy

Books
Sherr, Lorraine. *HIV and AIDS in Mothers and Babies.* Boston, MA: Blackwell Scientific Publications, 1991.

Drugs and alcohol in pregnancy

Videos
Drugs, Alcohol & Pregnancy, Human Relation Media, 1992.

Snowbabies – The Innocent Victims, Snowbabies, Inc., 1989.

Snowbabies II –The Generational Curse, Snowbabies, Inc., 1993.

Bedrest and preterm birth
Bedrest

Books
Johnston, Susan H., M.S.W. and Kraut, Deborah A., M.I.L.R. *Pregnancy Bedrest.* New York: Henry Holt and Company, Inc., 1990.

Isennock, Patricia, R.N., M.S. *Bedrest Before Baby.* Perry Hall, MD: Mustard Seed Publications, 1992.

Premature babies

Books
Ludington-Hoe, Susan, Ph.D. and Golant, Susan K. *Kangaroo Care, The Best You Can Do To Help Your Preterm Infant.* New York: Bantam Books, 1993.

Videos
Caring for Your NICU Baby, Brookes Publishing, 1994.

Introduction to the NICU, Brookes Publishing, 1994.

Pregnancy loss

Books
Diamond, Kathleen, M.D. *Motherhood After Miscarriage.* Holbrook, MA: Bob Adams, Inc., 1991.

Finnegan, Joanne. *Shattered Dreams–Lonely Choices.* Westport, CT: Bergin and Garvey, 1993.

Kohn, Ingrid, M.S.W. and Moffitt, Perry-Lynn. *A Silent Sorrow: Pregnancy Loss.* New York: Dell Publishing, 1992.

Shapiro, Constance Hoenk. *Infertility and Pregnancy Loss.* San Francisco, CA: Jossey-Bass Publishers, 1988.

Giving birth

Planning your birth

Books

Capacchione, Lucia, Ph.D., A.T.R., and Bardsley, Sandra, R.N., F.A.C.C.E. **Creating a Joyful Birth Experience**. New York: Fireside, 1994.

Kitzinger, Sheila, **Your Baby, Your Way: Making Pregnancy Decisions and Birth Plans**, New York: Panthoen. 1987

The process of labor and birth

Books

Balaskas, Jane. **Active Birth – The New Approach to Giving Birth Naturally.** Boston: Harvard Common Press, 1992.

McCullough, Stacy. **Your Special Baby – Real Lamaze Prepared Childbirth.** Newport Beach, California: Luckenbooth Press, 1993.

Videos

Having Your Baby – Lamaze, Parent Productions, 1985.

Special Delivery, Injoy Productions, 1988.

Welcome to the World – Three Birth Stories, Injoy Productions, 1992.

Focus on Labor & Delivery, WRS Group, Inc., 1990.

Gentle birth/water birth

Books

Harper, Barbara, R.N. **Gentle Birth Choices**. Rochester, VT: Healing Arts Press, 1994.

Napierala, Susanna. **Water Birth**. Westport, CT: Bergin and Garvey, 1994.

Odent, Michel, **Birth Reborn.** New York: Random House, 1984.

Birth assistants and doulas

Books

Placksin, Sally. **Mothering the New Mother**. New York: Newmarket Press, 1994.

Simkin, Penny, P.T. **The Birth Partner**. Boston: Harvard Common Press, 1989.

Managing labor pain

Books

Lieberman, Adrienne. **Easing Labor Pain, The Complete Guide to a More Comfortable and Rewarding Birth.** Boston: Harvard Common Press, 1992.

Cesarean

Books

Alvarez, Manuel, M.D. and Feiden, Karyn L. **Recovering from a Cesarean Section**. New York: Harper Paperbacks, 1993.

VBAC

Books

Flamm, Bruce, M.D. **Birth After Cesarean.** New York: Simon and Schuster, 1990.

Newborns and siblings

Newborns

Books

Klaus, M.D. and Klaus, Phyllis, M.Ed., C.S.W. **The Amazing Newborn**. Reading, MA: Addison-Wesley Publishing Co., Inc., 1985.

Stoppard, Miriam, M.D. **The First Weeks of Life**. New York: Dorling Kindersley, 1989.

Videos

The Circumcision Question, Wilbert Productions.

Sibling adjustment

Books

Kitzinger, Sheila. **Being Born**. New York: Grosset and Dunlap, 1986.

Videos

Hey, What About Me? KidVidz, 1987.

Postpartum

Books

Kleiman, Karen R., M.S.W. and Raskin, Valerie D., M.D. **This Isn't What I Expected**. New York: Bantam Books, 1994.

Lim, Robin. **After the Baby's Birth: A Woman's Way to Wellness**. Berkeley, CA: Celestial Arts, 1991.

Postpartum survival guide

Videos

Taking Care of Mom: A Guide to Postpartum, Lifecycle Productions, Inc., 1992.

Parenting and baby care

Parenting

Books

Alexander, Shoshana. *In Praise of Single Parents*. New York: Houghton Mifflin Co., 1994.

Bassoff, Evelyn S., Ph.D. *Mothering Ourselves*. New York: Penguin Group, 1991.

Eagan, Andrea Boroff. *The Newborn Mother*. New York: Henry Holt and Company, Inc., 1985.

Weisberg, Anne C. and Buckler, Carol A. *Everything a Working Mother Needs to Know*. New York: Doubleday, 1994.

Videos

Diapers and Delirium, Lifecycle Productions, Inc., 1987.

Sex, Love and Babies, Injoy Productions, 1993.

The Working Mom's Survival Guide, Xenejenex, Inc., 1990.

Baby care

Books

Carter, John Mack, et al. *The Good Housekeeping Illustrated Book of Pregnancy and Baby Care*. New York: Hearst Books, 1990.

Johnson, Robert V., M.D., et al. *Mayo Clinic Complete Book of Pregnancy and Baby's First Year*. New York: William Morrow and Co., Inc., 1994.

Lansky, Vicki, et al. *Complete Pregnancy and Baby Book*. Lincolnwood, IL: Publications International, Ltd., 1993.

Simkin, Penny, R.P.T., Whalley, Janet, R.N., B.S.N. and Keppler, Ann, R.N., M.N. *Pregnancy, Childbirth, and the Newborn*. New York: Meadowbrook Press, 1991.

Stoppard, Miriam, M.D. *Conception, Pregnancy and Birth*. New York: Dorling Kindersley, 1993.

Videos

Baby Talk, Polymorph Films, 1992.

Newborn Care, Cradle to Rock Productions, 1987.

Childproof, Home Safety Checklist, Promedion Productions, 1991.

Breastfeeding

Books

Mohrbacher, Nancy, I.B.C.L.C. and Stock, Julie, B.A. I.B.C.L.C. *The Breastfeeding Answer Book.* Franklin Park, IL: La Leche League International, 1993.

Gotch, Gwen. *Breastfeeding Pure and Simple.* Franklin Park, IL: La Leche League International, 1994.

Pfluke, Lillian. *Breastfeeding and the Active Woman.* Waco, TX: WRS Publishing, 1995.

La Leche League International. *The Womanly Art of Breastfeeding.* New York: Plume, The Penguin Group, 1991.

Huggins, Kathleen, RN, MS. *The Nursing Mother's Companion,* Boston: Harvard Common Press, 1990.

Behan, Eileen, RD. *Eat Well and Lose Weight While Breastfeeding,* New York: Villard Books, 1994.

Videos

Breastfeeding, A Special Relationship, Eagle Video Productions, 1991.

A Healthier Baby by Breastfeeding, Television Innovation Co., 1991.

Breastfeeding Your Baby, Medela, 1987.

Women's health and contraception

Books

Davidson, James, M.D. and Winebrenner, Jan. *In Touch With Your Breasts.* Waco, TX: WRS Publishing, 1995.

Hatcher, Robert, M.D., M.P.H., et al. *Contraceptive Technology.* New York: Irvington Publishers, Inc., 1995.

Videos

Women's Health Series, Medcom, Inc., 1993.
After Pregnancy
Breast Cancer
Contraception
Infertility
Menopause
Menstruation
Pregnancy
STDs

Bibliography

Alexander, Shoshana. *In Praise of Single Parents*. New York: Houghton Mifflin Co., 1994.

Alvarez, Manuel, M.D. and Feiden, Karyn L. *Recovering from a Cesarean Section*. New York: Harper Paperbacks, 1993.

Bassoff, Evelyn S., Ph.D. *Mothering Ourselves*. New York: Penguin Group, 1991.

Bolane, Jamie Eloise. *Life Unto Life*. Waco, TX: WRS Group, Inc., 1988.

Bolane, Jamie Eloise. *Breastfeeding Basics*. Waco, TX: WRS Group, Inc., 1988.

Capacchione, Lucia, Ph.D., A.T.R., and Bardsley, Sandra, R.N., F.A.C.C.E. *Creating a Joyful Birth Experience*. New York: Fireside, 1994.

Carter, John Mack, et al. *The Good Housekeeping Illustrated Book of Pregnancy and Baby Care*. New York: Hearst Books, 1990.

Curtis, Glade B., M.D., F.A.C.O.G. *Your Pregnancy Week by Week*. Tucson, AZ: Fisher Books, 1989.

Diamond, Kathleen, M.D. *Motherhood After Miscarriage*. Holbrook, MA: Bob Adams, Inc., 1991.

Duhnham, Carroll, et al. *Mamatoto, A Celebration of Birth*. New York: Viking Penguin, 1991.

Eagan, Andrea Boroff. *The Newborn Mother*. New York: Henry Holt and Company, Inc., 1985.

Eisenber, Arlene; Murkoff, Heidi E. and Hathaway, Sandee E. *What to Expect When You're Expecting*. New York: Workman Publishing, 1991.

Erick, Miriam, R.D., M.S. *No More Morning Sickness*. New York: The Penguin Group, 1993.

Finnegan, Joanne. *Shattered Dreams–Lonely Choices*. Westport, CT: Bergin and Garvey, 1993.

Flanagan, Geraldine Lux. *The First Nine Months of Life*. New York: Simon and Schuster, Inc., 1962.

Gardner, Joy. *Healing Yourself During Pregnancy*. Freedom, CA: The Crossing Press, 1987.

Harkness, Carla. *The Infertility Book*. Berkeley, CA: Celestial Arts, 1987.

Harper, Barbara, R.N. *Gentle Birth Choices*. Rochester, VT: Healing Arts Press, 1994.

Jacobs, Sandra and the American College of Nurse-Midwives. *Having Your Baby With a Nurse-Midwife*. New York: Hyperion, 1993.

Johnson, Robert V., M.D., et al. *Mayo Clinic Complete Book of Pregnancy and Baby's First Year*. New York: William Morrow and Co., Inc., 1994.

Johnston, Susan H., M.S.W. and Kraut, Deborah A., M.I.L.R. *Pregnancy Bedrest*. New York: Henry Holt and Company, Inc., 1990.

Kitzinger, Sheila. *The Complete Book of Pregnancy and Childbirth:* New York: Alfred A. Knopf, Inc., 1993.

Kitzinger, Sheila and Bailey, Vicky. *Pregnancy: Day by Day*. New York: Alfred A. Knopf, Inc., 1994.

Klaus, Marshall, M.D. and Klaus, Phyllis, M.Ed., C.S.W. *The Amazing Newborn*. Reading, MA: Addison-Wesley Publishing Co., Inc., 1985.

Kleiman, Karen R., M.S.W. and Raskin, Valerie D., M.D. *This Isn't What I Expected*. New York: Bantam Books, 1994.

Kohn, Ingrid, M.S.W. and Moffitt, Perry-Lynn. *A Silent Sorrow: Pregnancy Loss*. New York: Dell Publishing, 1992.

Lansky, Vicki, et al. *Complete Pregnancy and Baby Book*. Lincolnwood, IL: Publications International, Ltd., 1993.

Lewin, Benjamin. *Genes V*. Oxford: Oxford University Press, 1994.

Lim, Robin. *After the Baby's Birth: A Woman's Way to Wellness*. Berkeley, CA: Celestial Arts, 1991.

Ludington-Hoe, Susan, Ph.D. and Golant, Susan K. *Kangaroo Care, The Best You Can Do To Help Your Preterm Infant*. New York: Bantam Books, 1993.

Marshall, Connie, R.N. *The Expectant Father*. Citrus Heights, CA: Conmar Publishing, Inc., 1992.

Moore, Keith L., M.Sc., Ph.D. *The Developing Human 3rd Edition, Clinically Oriented Embryology*. Philadelphia, PA: W.B. Saunders Co., 1982.

Moore, Keith L., M.Sc., Ph.D. *Essentials of Human Embryology*. Toronto: B.C. Decker Inc., 1988.

Napierala, Susanna. *Water Birth*. Westport, CT: Bergin and Garvey, 1994.

Nilsson, Lennart and Hamberger, Lars. *A Child Is Born*. New York: Delacorte Press/Seymor Lawrence, 1990.

Peterson, Gayle, Ph.D. *An Easier Childbirth*. Berkeley, CA: Shadow and Light Publications, 1993.

Placksin, Sally. *Mothering the New Mother*. New York: Newmarket Press, 1994.

Poole, Catherine M. and Parr, Elizabeth A., C.N.M. *Choosing a Nurse-Midwife*. New York: John Wiley and Sons, Inc., 1994.

Rothman, Barbara Katz, et al. *The Encyclopedia of Childbearing*. New York: Henry Holt and Company, Inc., 1993.

Rowe, Bruce M. and Stein, Philip L. *Physical Anthropology*. New York: McGraw-Hill, Inc., 1993.

Russell, Peter J. *Genetics 3rd Edition*. New York: HarperCollins Publishers Inc., 1992.

Samuels, Mike, M.D., and Samuels, Nancy. *The Well Pregnancy Book*. New York: Fireside, 1986.

Shapiro, Constance Hoenk. *Infertility and Pregnancy Loss*. San Francisco, CA: Jossey-Bass Publishers, 1988.

Shapiro, Harriet Roberts, R.N., A.C.C.E., et al. *The Lamaze Ready-Reference Guide for Labor and Birth*. 1990. Washington DC: Washington DC Chapter – A.S.P.O./ Lamaze, 1990.

Shapiro, Jerrold Lee, Ph.D. *When Men Are Pregnant*. New York: Dell Publishing, 1987.

Sherr, Lorraine. *HIV and AIDS in Mothers and Babies*. Boston, MA: Blackwell Scientific Publications, 1991.

Simkin, Penny, R.P.T.; Whalley, Janet, R.N., B.S.N. and Keppler, Ann, R.N., M.N. *Pregnancy, Childbirth, and the Newborn*. New York: Meadowbrook Press, 1991.

Stillerman, Elaine, L.M.T. *Mother Massage*. New York: Dell Publishing, 1992.

Stoppard, Miriam, M.D. *Conception, Pregnancy and Birth*. New York: Dorling Kindersley, 1993.

Stoppard, Miriam, M.D. *The New Pregnancy and Birth Book*. New York: Dorling Kindersley, 1991.

Stukane, Eileen. *The Dream Worlds of Pregnancy*. Barrytown, NY: Station Hill Press, Inc.,1985.

Sussman, John R., M.D., and Levitt, B. Blake. *Before You Conceive, The Complete Prepregnancy Guide*. New York: Bantam Books, 1989.

Ting, Rosalind Y., M.D., M.P.H., et al. *The Complete Mothercare Manual*. New York: Fireside, 1987.

Van Der Meer, Antonia. *Great Expectations*. New York: Dell Publishing, 1993.

Visscher, Harrison C., M.D., F.A.C.O.G., et al. *Planning for Pregnancy, Birth, and Beyond*. New York: The Penguin Group, 1990.

Weisberg, Anne C. and Buckler, Carol A. *Everything a Working Mother Needs to Know*. New York: Doubleday, 1994.

Resource organizations

General maternal and child health

American College of Nurse-Midwives
818 Connecticut Ave. NW,
Suite 900
Washington, DC 20006
(202) 728-9860

American College of Obstetricians and Gynecologists
409 12th St. SW
Washington, DC 20024-2188
(202) 638-5577

March of Dimes Birth Defects Foundation National Office
1275 Mamaroneck Ave.
White Plains, NY 10605
(914) 428-7100

National Council for Adoption
1930 17th St., NW
Washington, DC 20009
(202) 328-1200

National Women's Health Network
514 10th St., NW, Suite 400
Washington, DC 20004
(202) 347-1140

Planned Parenthood Federation of America
810 Seventh Ave.
New York, NY 10019
(212) 541-7800

Birth centers

Maternity Center Association (MCA)
48 East 92nd St.
New York, NY 10128
(212) 777-5000

National Association of Childbearing Centers (NACC)
3123 Gottschall Rd.
Perkiomenville, PA 18074
(215) 234-8068

Midwifery

American College of Nurse-Midwives
818 Connecticut Ave. NW, Suite 900
Washington, DC 20006
(202) 728-9860

Birth assistants and doulas

Doulas of North America (DONA)
1100 23rd Ave. East
Seattle, WA 98112
(206) 324-5440

High-risk pregnancy

Access to Respite Care and Help (ARCH)
National Resource Center for Crisis Nurseries and Respite Care Services
800 Eastowne Drive, Suite 105
Chapel Hill, NC 27514
(800) 473-1727

DES Action U.S.A.
1615 Broadway, Suite 510
Oakland, CA 94612
(510) 465-4011

Group B Strep Association
P.O. Box 16515
Chapel Hill, NC 27516
(919) 932-5344

March of Dimes Birth Defects Foundation
1275 Mamaroneck Ave.
White Plains, NY 10605
(914) 428-7100
Parent-to-Parent
University of Utah Hospital
50 North Medical Drive, Rm 2553
Salt Lake City, UT 84132
(801) 581-2098

Sidelines National Support Network
P.O. Box 1808
Laguna Beach, CA 92652
(949) 497-2265

Bedrest in pregnancy

The Confinement Line
P.O. Box 1609
Springfield, VA 22151
(703) 941-7183

National Organization of Mothers of Twins Club
P.O. Box 23188
Albuquerque, NM 87192-1188
(505) 275-0955

Sidelines National Support Network
2805 Park Place
Laguna Beach, CA 92651
(949) 497-2265

Triplet Connection
P.O. Box 99571
Stockton, CA 95209
(209) 474-0885

Pregnancy and infant loss

The Compassionate Friends
P.O. Box 3696
Oak Brook, IL 60522-3696
(630) 990-0010

Sudden infant death syndrome

Pregnancy and Infant Loss Center
1421 E. Wayzata Blvd., Suite 30
Wayzata, MN 55391
(612) 473-9372

Resolve Through Sharing Bereavement Services Lutheran Hospital–La Crosse
1910 South Ave.
La Crosse, WI 54601
(608) 791-4747
(800) 362-9567 ext. 4747

Share
St. John's Hospital
800 E. Carpenter
Springfield, IL 62769
(217) 525-5675

Sudden Infant Death Syndrome (SIDS) Alliance
1314 Bedford Ave., Suite 210
Baltimore, MD 21208
(800) 221-7437

Birth education

American Academy of Husband-Coached Childbirth
P.O. Box 5224
Sherman Oaks, CA 91413
(818) 788-6662

American Society of Psychoprophylaxis in Obstetrics (ASPO Lamaze)
1200 19th St. NW, Suite 300
Washington, DC 20036-2412
(800) 368-4404

International Childbirth Education Association (ICEA)
P.O. Box 20048
Minneapolis, MN 55420-0048
(612) 854-8660

Homebirth

Informed Homebirth/Informed Birth and Parenting
P.O. Box 3675
Ann Arbor, MI 48106
(734) 662-6857

International Association of Parents and Professionals for Safe Alternatives in Childbirth (NAPSAC)
Route 1, Box 646
Marble Hill, MO 63764
(573) 238-2010

Cesarean & VBAC

Cesarean Support, Education, and Concern (C/SEC)
22 Forest Road
Framingham, MA 01701
(508) 877-8266

International Cesarean Awareness Network, Inc. (ICAN)
1304 Kingsdale Ave.
Redondo Beach, CA 90278
(310) 542-6400

Circumcision

National Organization of Circumcision Information Resource Centers (NOCIRC)
P.O. Box 2512
San Anselmo, CA 94979
(415) 488-9883

Postpartum adjustment

After the Stork
6 San Tomas
Rancho Santa Margarita, CA 92688
(949) 589-4311

National Association of Postpartum Care Services (NAPCS)
P.O. Box 1020
Edmonds, WA 98020

Postpartum Adjustment Support Services (PASS—Canada)
P.O. Box 7282
Oakville, Ontario L6J 6L6
Canada
(905) 844-9009

Postpartum Assistance for Mothers (PAM)
PAM East Bay
P.O. Box 20513
Castro Valley, CA 94546
(510) 727-4610

Postpartum Support International
927 N. Kellogg Ave.
Santa Barbara, CA 93111
(805) 967-7636

Parenting

The Fatherhood Project
Bank St. College of Education
610 W. 112th St.
New York, NY 10025
(212) 337-0934

Single parents

Single Mothers by Choice (SMC)
P.O. Box 1642
Gracie Square Station
New York, NY 10028
(212) 988-0993

Twins

Center for Study of Multiple Births
333 E. Superior #464
Chicago, IL 60611
(312) 266-9093

International Twins Association, Inc.
6898 Channel Road
Minneapolis, MN 55432
(612) 571-3022

National Organization of Mothers of Twins Clubs
P.O. Box 23188
Albuquerque, NM 87192-1188
(505) 275-0955

Breastfeeding

Infant Feeding Action Coalition (INFACT)
10 Trinity Square
Toronto, Ontario M5G 1B1
Canada
(416) 595-9819

International Lactation Consultant Association (ILCA)
201 Brown Ave.
Evanston, IL 60202-3601
(919) 787-5181

La Leche League of Canada
18C Industrial Drive, Box 29
Chesterville, Ontario KOC1HO
Canada
(613) 448-1842

La Leche League International (LLLI)
1400 N. Meecham Rd.
Schaumberg, IL 60173
(708) 519-7730
(800) LA LECHE

Lactation Institute
16430 Ventura Blvd., Suite 303
Encino, CA 91436
(818) 995-1913

Genetics

Alliance of Genetic Support Groups
35 Wisconsin Circle, Suite 440
Chevy Chase, MD 20815
(800) 336-4363

American Society of Andrology
74 New Montgomery St., Suite 230
San Francisco, CA 94105
(415) 764-4822

March of Dimes Birth Defect Foundation
Professional Education Department
1275 Mamaroneck Ave.
White Plains, NY 10605
(914) 428-7100

Fertility and infertility

Endometriosis Association
8585 North 76th Place
Milwaukee, WI 53223
(800) 992-3636 (US)
(800) 426-2363 (Canada)

Resolve
1310 Broadway
Somerville, MA 02144-1731
(617) 623-1156 – Main number
(617) 623-0744 – Helpline

Special-needs children

ARC National Headquarters
500 E. Border, Suite 300
Arlington, TX 76010
(817) 261-6003

Cleft Palate Foundation
104 S. Estes Dr., Suite 204
Chapel Hill, NC 27514
(800) 24-CLEFT

Federation for Children with Special Needs
95 Berkeley St., Suite 104
Boston, MA 02116
(617) 482-2915

National Information Center for Children and Youth with Handicaps
P.O. Box 1492
Washington, DC 20013
(800) 695-0285

Mothers at home

FEMALE (Formerly Employed Mothers At the Leading Edge)
P.O. Box 31
Elmhurst, IL 60126
(630) 941-3553

Mothers at Home
8310A Old Courthouse Road
Vienna, VA 22182
(703) 827-5903
(800) 783-4666

Mothers' Home Business Network
P.O. Box 423A
East Meadow, NY 11554
(516) 997-7394

Welfare Warriors Voice Newspaper
2711 W. Michigan
Milwaukee, WI 53208
(414) 342-6662

Mothers working outside the home

9 to 5 National Association of Working Women
614 Superior Ave., NW
Cleveland, OH 44113
(216) 566-9308
(800) 522-0925

Catalyst
250 Park Ave S., 5th Floor
New York, NY 10003
(212) 514-7600

Minnesota Vocational Education Work & Family Institute
Hennepin Technical College
1820 N. Xenium Lane
Plymouth, MN 55441
(612) 550-7155

National Council of Jewish Women Work/Family Project
53 West 23rd St.
New York, NY 10010
(212) 645-4048

New Ways to Work
785 Market St., Suite 950
San Francisco, CA 94103
(415) 995-9860

Work and Family Clearinghouse
U.S. Department of Labor, Women's Bureau
200 Constitution Ave., NW
Washington, DC 20210
(800) 827-5335
(202) 219-4486

Work/Family Directions, Inc.
928 Commonwealth Ave. West
Boston, MA 02215-1204
(617) 264-3200

Workplace Options
109 South Bloodworth St.
Raleigh, NC 27601
(800) 699-8011
(919) 834-6506

kripalu
summer
salads,
sandwiches,
and soups

from Executive Chef
Deb Morgan

exploring the yoga of life.

table of contents

on the cover: gazpacho, Greek salad with feta, and chickpea of the sea sandwich

introduction

Salads, Sandwiches, and Summer Soups

Delicious, Nutritious, and Easy!

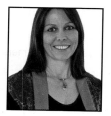 With this edition of our recipe book series, we break out of our normal meal format to highlight some of the lighter, simple, individual recipes we offer during the summer.

As the temperatures rise and the gardens and farmer's markets burst with produce, it's time to get creative with vegetables. At Kripalu, we're lucky to have great relationships with several local farms that supply us with an abundance of local lettuces, kale and chard, greens beans and snap peas, tomatoes, and herbs, plus root vegetables and squashes that we enjoy later in the season.

In addition to our extensive salad bar, we also feature a wonderful sandwich bar, which offers a rotating menu of sandwich fixings, such as chicken salads that include fresh mint, tarragon, or curry, or our crunchy Tuna

Apple Walnut Salad. Our vegetarian offerings include a simple hummus and Kripalu signature dishes such as our Chickpea of the Sea and our Carrot Sunflower Spread.

This edition also offers you 20 of our favorite salads, from 100 percent raw creations to a classic Greek salad to a variety of cold salads that feature whole grains, beans, and pasta.

And what salad book would be complete without healthful salad dressings, like the all-time guest favorite, the Kripalu House Dressing?

As a bonus, we've included four of our favorite iced teas to help keep you cool and energized throughout the summer. Our guests can't get enough of it: In the summer, we make more than 60 gallons of iced tea a day!

And as always, we've included words of wisdom from some of Kripalu's teachers. This time, we hear from Aruni Nan

Futuronsky on mindful eating, learn nutritional tips from Annie B. Kay, and get gardening inspiration from John Bagnulo.

I do hope the beautiful photographs inspire you to race out to your local farmer's market (or your own garden), pick up a basket full of vegetables, and create an amazing treat!

I end with our Kripalu Kitchen motto to serve you as a guide on your cooking and eating endeavors: Quality. Choice. Intention. Start with quality ingredients, choose the foods that are right for you and your health, and bring an intention of love to the entire process.

Remember, when we cook love, we live love.

Executive Chef Deb Morgan
Kripalu Center for Yoga & Health

acknowledgments

"The whole world is one family." This key message from Swami Kripalu came to me when I thought of all the people I need to acknowledge for their contributions to this book. Dedication to wholesome, delicious food has served as a wonderful meeting place for many. So thank you to the guests and staff who grace our Dining Hall each day and give us feedback on our cuisine. Thank you to the farmers whose love of food nourishes us all on many levels. Thank you to the entire Kripalu Kitchen staff for sharing the light that is your life with me every day.

Special appreciation goes to my hardworking recipe testers for this issue: our kitchen intern, Stephanie Michalak, and Cheryl Holmes, whose devotion to natural foods has been offered so lovingly to this project.

And to Jeremy Smith, our talented chef de cuisine, who can cut vegetables so much faster then I can, but lets me be the Executive Chef anyway. Thank you to our Marketing and Communications Department's patient staff of editors and organizers, and artistic wiz, Elena Erber. Thank you to Jennifer May and Jessica Bard for bringing the beauty of the Kripalu cuisine to these pages with sumptuous photography.

And thank you to Swami Kripalu for the inspiration that started it all for me almost 25 years ago. Om Shanti.

fresh herbs

Parsley, rosemary, thyme, cilantro, mint, basil, oregano, lavender … the list of herbs we love and their many uses is endless. In the Kripalu Kitchen, we use fresh herbs year-round, but when summer's warm weather comes, their appeal is even stronger. Fresh herbs add an uplifting layer of flavor and an enlivening aroma. Once you get in the habit of buying fresh herbs (or better yet, growing them yourself) you will find that they are hard to cook without.

Here are some tips on how to use and preserve your fresh herbs this summer:

1. Rinse large leaf herbs, such as parsley, cilantro, and basil, very well. These leaves are large enough that little bits of sand or dirt often get stuck to them.

2. Store fresh herbs upright in the refrigerator with their stems in water. This will ensure that they stay fresh longer—simply change the water every few days.

3. Large leaf herbs can be blended with olive oil and a pinch of salt or garlic to make a great flavor additive to any dish. Store in the refrigerator for the short-term, or place them in an ice cube tray in the freezer for longer-term storage. Just pop out a "flavor cube" when needed.

4. The safest way to infuse oils with any herb is to lightly simmer the herbs in oil for five minutes, then strain the oil through a cheesecloth and store them in the refrigerator.

5. Make a refreshing drink by adding a few fresh herbs (plus cucumber and lemon) to a pitcher of water. It's much more refreshing than plain water.

6. Enliven your black, green, or rooibos iced tea by steeping it with fresh herbs. My favorite recipe of the season is our Lavender Black Tea with Honey (see page 54).

salads

American salads have come a long way. We no longer have to settle for iceberg lettuce topped with pale tomatoes and Thousand Island dressing. Instead, a bounty of spring mixes, baby spinach, arugula, leaf lettuces, and crispy romaine have made appearances as side salads and have even taken center stage as entrees. And recently, salads made with an array of vegetables combined with grains, beans, or pasta have taken up residence on many menus.

Of course, freshness counts when it comes to salad greens and vegetables, as does organic. So choose local, unsprayed produce whenever possible. The most important thing to remember is to experiment: Feel free to mix and match ingredients as you try out these recipes.

vegetable salads

The greens and add-ins in these versatile salads are all interchangeable. If feta cheese isn't your thing, make our Greek salad without it, or add in cubes of tofu. If you don't eat bacon but want to try the Arugula, Date, Almond, and Bacon Salad, go with vegetarian tempeh bacon or crispy toasted pumpkin seeds. Each of these recipes offers a multitude of flavor profiles based on the ingredients you choose, so have fun with it!

arugula, date, almond, and bacon salad with baked goat cheese

Serves 4

for pecan-thyme goat cheese
1/3 cup roasted pecans, finely chopped
1 teaspoons minced fresh thyme
Pinch of sea salt

for parsley-pepper goat cheese
1/3 cup minced fresh parsley
1/8 teaspoon coarsely ground black pepper
Pinch of sea salt

8 ounces fresh goat cheese

for the salad
8 cups arugula
3 tablespoons extra-virgin olive oil
2 teaspoons balsamic vinegar
Pinch of sea salt
1/3 cup sliced dried dates
1/4 cup toasted slivered almonds
1/2 cup cooked turkey bacon or Fakin' Bacon™ (tempeh product), chopped into small pieces

Preheat oven to 350 degrees. Mix together the pecan-thyme ingredients in a small bowl and set aside. Mix together the parsley-pepper ingredients in a small bowl and set aside.

Divide goat cheese into 8 pieces (about 1 ounce each) and form into balls. Place 4 cheese balls into the pecan-thyme mixture and gently roll until each is coated. Repeat using the parsley-pepper mixture and remaining cheese balls.

Place the cheese balls on a baking sheet. You can leave them round or flatten each ball slightly if desired. Bake until warmed through but not melted, about 3 to 4 minutes. Alternatively, goat cheese balls may be served chilled.

While the cheese balls are heating, combine the arugula, olive oil, vinegar, and salt in a large mixing bowl and toss thoroughly. Divide the dressed arugula between 4 plates and arrange the dates, almonds, and bacon on top of each. Place two baked goat cheese balls on each plate and serve immediately.

arugula, date, almond, and bacon salad with baked goat cheese

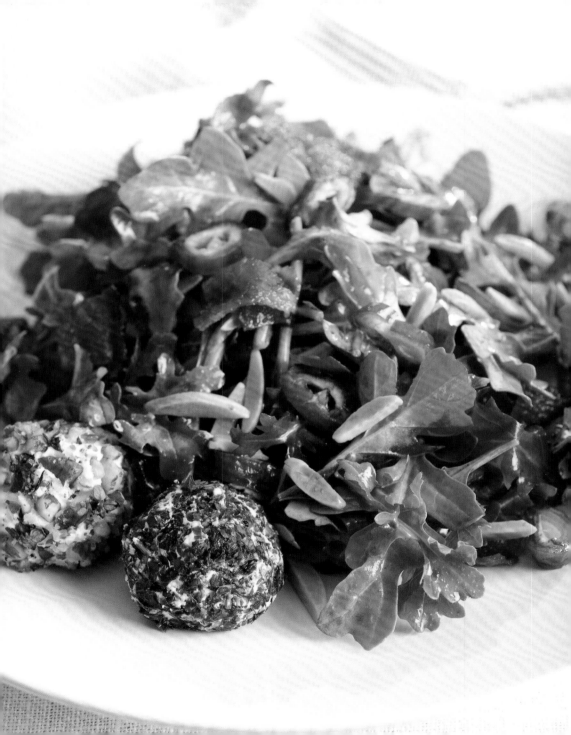

greek salad with feta

Serves 4

for the dressing
5 tablespoons extra-virgin olive oil
1 tablespoon red wine vinegar
1 teaspoon fresh lemon juice
1 tablespoon minced garlic
1 tablespoon sliced scallion
1/2 teaspoon dried basil
1/2 teaspoon dried thyme
1/2 teaspoon sea salt
Pinch of black pepper

for the salad
6 cups shredded romaine lettuce
1/2 cup grape tomatoes, cut in half
1/2 cup diced cucumber
1/2 cup diced red onion
1/2 cup cubed feta cheese
1/4 cup kalamata olives, pitted and cut in half

Whisk the dressing ingredients together in a large mixing bowl. Add the salad ingredients and toss together until coated with the dressing. Serve immediately.

caesar salad deluxe

Serves 4

for the dressing
1 teaspoon Dijon mustard
2 tablespoons all-natural mayonnaise or
    Veganaise™ (egg-less mayonnaise)
3 tablespoons extra-virgin olive oil
1 tablespoon fresh lemon juice
1 teaspoon minced garlic
2 tablespoons grated Parmesan cheese
1/4 teaspoon Worcestershire sauce
1/4 teaspoon sea salt

for the salad
4 cups shredded romaine lettuce
4 cups spring mix lettuce

for the croutons
1 cup fresh bread cubes (1/2-inch pieces)
1 teaspoon finely minced garlic
2 tablespoons extra-virgin olive oil
Pinch of sea salt
Pinch of black pepper

Preheat oven to 325 degrees. Heat the oil in a large sauté pan over medium heat. Add the garlic and cook for 30 seconds. Add the bread cubes, sprinkle with salt and pepper, and sauté for about 1 minute, tossing until coated. Transfer seasoned bread cubes to a baking sheet and bake until golden brown, 5 to 8 minutes. Set aside to cool.

Whisk the dressing ingredients together in a large mixing bowl. Add the salad ingredients and croutons and toss together until coated with the dressing. Serve immediately.

edamame salad

Serves 4

for the salad

8 cups chopped green leaf lettuce
1 cup frozen shelled edamame (soybeans),
    thawed
1/2 cup sliced radishes
1/2 cup grated daikon radish

Ume Scallion Dressing (see page 24 for recipe)

Combine the salad ingredients in a large mixing bowl. Add 1/4 cup of the Ume Scallion Dressing and toss until well mixed. Taste and add more dressing if desired. Serve immediately.

waldorf salad

Serves 4

3 apples, cored
1 tablespoon fresh lemon juice
2 stalks celery, chopped
1/2 cup chopped walnuts
1/4 cup raisins (or other dried fruit)
1/2 cup Veganaise™ (egg-less mayonnaise)
1 1/2 teaspoons mustard (preferably stone-ground)
1/8 teaspoon sea salt
Black pepper to taste

Dice the apples and place in large mixing bowl. Sprinkle with the lemon juice and toss to prevent browning. Stir in the celery, walnuts, and raisins.

Combine the Veganaise, mustard, salt, and pepper in a small bowl. Add to the apple mixture and stir well to combine. Serve chilled.

spinach egg salad

Serves 4

for the dressing

2 tablespoons finely minced shallot
1 teaspoon apple cider vinegar
1 tablespoon champagne vinegar
2 tablespoons agave nectar
1/4 cup extra-virgin olive oil

for the salad

8 cups baby spinach
4 hard-boiled eggs, sliced
1/2 cup half-moon-sliced red onion
1/2 cup half-moon-sliced cucumber
1/4 cup toasted pumpkin seeds

Whisk the dressing ingredients together in a large mixing bowl. (If desired, warm dressing lightly and return to bowl.) Add the spinach and toss together until coated with the dressing. To serve, sprinkle or arrange the eggs, red onion, cucumber, and pumpkin seeds on top of the spinach. Serve immediately.

sunny arame salad

Serves 4

for the salad
1 1/2 cups dried arame seaweed
1/2 cup green beans, sliced lengthwise
1/2 cup diced red bell pepper
1/3 cup toasted sunflower seeds

for the dressing
1 tablespoon tamari
1 teaspoon toasted sesame oil
1 teaspoon brown rice vinegar
1 teaspoon ginger juice* (optional)

Soak arame in warm water until softened, about 5 minutes. Drain thoroughly and set aside.

Fill a medium sauce pot half full with water and bring to a boil. Add the green beans and cook until tender crisp, 1 to 2 minutes. Drain and cool.

Whisk the dressing ingredients together in a large mixing bowl. Add the drained arame, cooked green beans, red pepper, and sunflower seeds and toss together until thoroughly blended. The salad can be served immediately or refrigerated for several hours before serving.

*To make your own ginger juice, grate a piece of ginger on the finest setting of your grater or use a grater specifically designed for ginger. Place grated ginger in a piece of cheesecloth and squeeze to extract juice.

carrot pineapple salad

Serves 4

for the dressing
2 tablespoons minced fresh mint
2 tablespoons minced fresh cilantro
2 tablespoons extra-virgin olive oil
2 tablespoons fresh lime juice
1 tablespoon honey
1/4 teaspoon sea salt
2 scallions, sliced

for the salad
3 cups grated carrot
1 cup canned pineapple chunks, drained
1/2 cup toasted coconut flakes
1/4 cup toasted pumpkin seeds

Whisk the dressing ingredients together in a large mixing bowl. Add the salad ingredients and toss together until thoroughly blended. Refrigerate for several hours before serving. Serve cold or at room temperature.

nutrional wisdom
summertime phytonutrients
Annie B. Kay, MS, RD, PYT, integrative dietitian

Summer is perfect for opening our senses to all that's fresh and local. Choosing produce grown close to home yields great taste, supports your community's farmers and economy, and cultivates a more direct connection to the earth. Nothing is more local than the herbs and greens you grow yourself. Greens are chock full of phytonutrients, plant compounds that provide a range of anti-bacterial and anti-inflammatory benefits, as well as support the body's natural detoxification process. Even if you're not a gardener, you can still get a huge nutritional bang for your effort-filled buck by planting a few parsley, cilantro, or basil seeds in a window box.

Scientists are learning more about the power of phytonutrients every day. A single piece of fruit or serving of vegetable may contain hundreds or even thousands of different kinds, and the complex phytonutrient profiles of simple-seeming plants reminds us of the complexity of nature and of life itself. The role these nutrients play in health—if and how they synergize with other nutrients, and the interplay between them and our environments and lifestyle choices—are all active areas of research.

It's clear that scientists are discovering what yogis have known all along: Fresh, local herbs and produce carry the essence of health. Let's enjoy the taste of what summer offers us now.

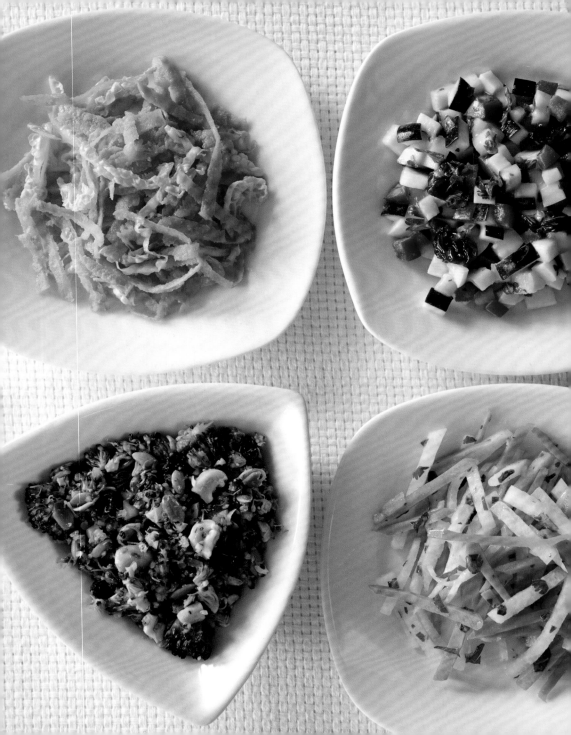

100% raw salads

There are many wonderful things about 100 percent raw salads. They burst with flavor —you can really taste the fresh ingredients—and they're quick and easy to create. As an added bonus, they won't raise the temperature in your kitchen on a hot summer day. I especially love to play around with jicama as an ingredient. Try it out; you may love how it adds a light, crispy, subtly sweet flavor.

raw spring fling salad

Serves 4

for the dressing
3 tablespoons extra-virgin olive oil
1 tablespoon Dijon mustard
1 1/2 teaspoons apple cider vinegar
1/8 teaspoon sea salt

for the salad
1 1/2 cups diced zucchini
1 1/2 cups diced summer squash
1/2 cup diced red bell pepper
2 tablespoons minced fresh parsley
1/4 cup dried cherries

Whisk the dressing ingredients together in a large mixing bowl. Add the salad ingredients and toss together until thoroughly blended. The salad can be served immediately or refrigerated for several hours before serving.

raw broccoli salad

Serves 4

for the dressing
3 tablespoons extra-virgin olive oil
2 tablespoons finely minced red onion
1 tablespoon apple cider vinegar
1 1/2 teaspoons raw honey
1/2 teaspoon Dijon mustard
1/4 teaspoon sea salt

for the salad
2 1/2 cups finely chopped broccoli florets
1/4 cup sunflower seeds
1/4 cup raisins
1/4 cup chopped raw cashews

Whisk the dressing ingredients together in a large mixing bowl. Add the salad ingredients and toss together until thoroughly blended. The salad can be served immediately or refrigerated for several hours before serving.

clockwise from top left: raw sweet potato salad, raw spring fling salad, raw jicama salad, raw broccoli salad

raw jicama salad

Serves 4

for the dressing
3 tablespoons extra-virgin olive oil
2 tablespoons fresh lime juice
1 tablespoon raw honey
1 tablespoon minced fresh cilantro
1/8 teaspoon sea salt
Pinch of ground cumin

for the salad
3 1/2 cups matchstick-cut jicama
1 1/2 cups matchstick-cut carrots

Whisk the dressing ingredients together in a large mixing bowl. Add the salad ingredients and toss together until thoroughly blended. The salad can be served immediately or refrigerated for several hours before serving.

raw sweet potato salad

Serves 4

for the dressing
1/4 cup extra-virgin olive oil
2 tablespoons fresh lime juice
1/8 teaspoon sea salt

for the salad
3 cups grated sweet potatoes, peeled
1 cup shredded napa cabbage

Whisk the dressing ingredients together in a large mixing bowl. Add the salad ingredients and toss together until thoroughly blended. The salad can be served immediately or refrigerated for several hours before serving.

grain, bean, and noodle salads

Although each of these salads offers a unique flavor combination, they all share one convenient attribute: They can be made from leftovers! Grains, beans, and pasta expand so much when they cook that you often have extra on hand. I like to put the leftover amount to good use in a hearty salad. Of course, fresh grains, beans, and pasta are fine to use too, and if you cook them just for the salad, be sure to let them come to room temperature before assembling the salad. This will ensure that your raw vegetables and toasted seeds maintain their crispness.

strawberry rice salad

Serves 4

for the dressing
1/4 cup Veganaise™ (egg-less mayonnaise)
2 teaspoons champagne vinegar
2 teaspoons honey
1 teaspoon apple cider vinegar
Pinch of sea salt

for the salad
2 cups cooked white basmati rice
1/2 cup diced mango (fresh or frozen and thawed)
1/2 cup sliced fresh strawberries
1/4 cup sliced dried dates
1/4 cup sliced celery

Whisk the dressing ingredients together in a large mixing bowl. Add the salad ingredients and gently stir until just blended. This salad is best served at room temperature.

brown rice sushi salad

Serves 4

1 tablespoon tamari
1 teaspoon brown rice vinegar
1 teaspoon umeboshi plum paste*
2 cups cooked short-grain brown rice
1/2 cup grated carrot
3 scallions, sliced
1/2 cup finely diced cucumber
2 tablespoons toasted black or white sesame seeds
1 toasted nori sheet, cut into 4 strips

Combine the tamari, brown rice vinegar, and umeboshi paste in a large mixing bowl. Add the remaining ingredients, except the nori, and stir well until thoroughly blended. Serve in individual bowls, each garnished with a strip of nori. This salad is best served at room temperature.

*Umeboshi plum paste, made from pickled Japanese plums and red shiso leaves, is dark pink and has a tangy, salty taste. It is available in the Asian section of most natural-foods stores.

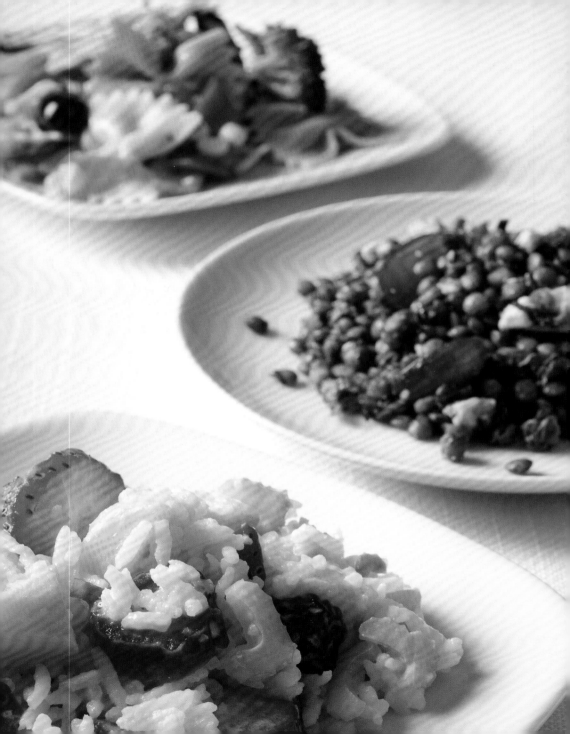

quinoa tabouli salad

Serves 4

1/2 cup quinoa
3/4 cup plus 2 tablespoons water
2 cups minced fresh parsley
1/4 cup fresh lemon juice
1/4 cup finely diced cucumber
1/4 cup diced tomato, drained
3 tablespoons extra-virgin olive oil
2 tablespoons minced fresh mint
Pinch of sea salt
Pinch of black pepper

Preheat oven to 350 degrees. Thoroughly rinse quinoa, drain well, and spread out on a baking sheet. Bake until quinoa starts to brown, stirring occasionally, about 10 minutes.

Place toasted quinoa in a sauce pot with the water. Bring to a boil then reduce heat, cover, and simmer for 10 minutes. Remove from heat, keep covered, and let rest for 10 minutes. Fluff quinoa with a fork and spread on platter to cool.

Transfer the cooled quinoa to a large mixing bowl. Add the remaining ingredients and stir gently until thoroughly combined. Serve at room temperature.

summer rice and bean salad

Serves 4

for the dressing
3 tablespoons extra-virgin olive oil
2 tablespoons balsamic vinegar
2 tablespoons minced fresh parsley
1 teaspoon minced fresh oregano
1 teaspoon minced fresh basil
1 teaspoon minced fresh rosemary
1/2 teaspoon sea salt
Pinch of black pepper

for the salad
3 cups cooked long-grain rice
1 15-ounce can garbanzo beans (chickpeas),
    drained or 1 1/4 cups cooked garbanzo beans
1/2 red bell pepper, small diced
1/2 green bell pepper, small diced
1/2 cup diced tomatoes
1/4 cup grated carrot
1/4 cup toasted sunflower seeds
1 stalk celery, small diced
2 scallions, sliced

Whisk the dressing ingredients together in a large mixing bowl. Add the salad ingredients and stir gently until thoroughly blended. This salad is best served at room temperature.

front to back: strawberry rice salad, french lentil salad, italian pasta salad

mexican black bean salad

Serves 2

for the dressing
2 1/2 tablespoons extra-virgin olive oil
2 tablespoons minced fresh cilantro
2 tablespoons fresh lemon juice
1 1/2 teaspoons umeboshi plum vinegar
1 teaspoon agave nectar
1 teaspoon ground cumin
Pinch of sea salt

for the salad
1 15-ounce can black beans, drained, or
   1 1/4 cups cooked black beans
1/2 cup fresh corn, cooked and cooled
1/4 cup grated carrot
1 stalk celery, chopped
2 tablespoons minced fresh parsley

Whisk the dressing ingredients together in a large mixing bowl. Add the salad ingredients and stir gently until thoroughly blended. The salad can be served immediately or refrigerated for several hours before serving.

french lentil salad

Serves 4

1 cup French lentils
2 1/2 cups water
1 bay leaf
1/2 cup red or green grapes, cut into quarters
1/4 cup feta cheese, cut into small cubes
1/4 cup extra-virgin olive oil
2 tablespoons minced red onion
2 tablespoons minced fresh mint
2 tablespoons minced fresh cilantro
1 tablespoon balsamic vinegar
1 teaspoon minced garlic
1/2 teaspoon sea salt

Place lentils in a sauce pot with the water and bay leaf. Bring to a boil, then reduce heat, partially cover, and simmer until lentils are soft but still intact, 20 to 30 minutes. Drain well. Remove the bay leaf and spread on platter to cool.

Transfer the cooled lentils to a large mixing bowl. Add the remaining ingredients and stir gently until thoroughly blended. Serve chilled or at room temperature.

cold sesame noodles

Serves 4

for the dressing
1/3 cup plus 1 tablespoon water
1/3 cup peanut butter
2 1/2 tablespoons tamari
2 tablespoons toasted sesame seeds
1 1/2 tablespoons rice vinegar
1 tablespoon agave nectar
1 tablespoon tahini
1 teaspoon toasted sesame oil
3/4 teaspoon bottled hot sauce or
    chili sauce, to taste

for the salad
3/4 pound udon noodles
1 cup matchstick-cut cucumber
2 tablespoons minced fresh cilantro
1 scallion, sliced

Whisk the dressing ingredients together in a large mixing bowl and set aside.

Cook noodles according to package directions. Drain and rinse under cold water. Add the noodles to the dressing and toss until well combined. Add the cucumber and cilantro and gently fold until thoroughly combined. Serve immediately, garnished with the scallion.

italian pasta salad

Serves 4

for the dressing
5 tablespoons extra-virgin olive oil
3 tablespoons minced fresh parsley
2 tablespoons sherry vinegar
2 tablespoons minced fresh basil
1 tablespoon minced garlic
2 teaspoons fresh lemon juice
1/4 teaspoon sea salt

for the salad
1/2 pound bowtie pasta
1 cup bite-size broccoli florets*
1 cup diagonally sliced snow peas*
1/2 cup fresh corn, cooked and cooled
1/2 cup pitted kalamata olives, cut in half

Canned tuna fish, drained (optional)
Crumbled or diced feta, goat, or sharp cheddar
    cheese (optional)

Whisk the dressing ingredients together in a large mixing bowl and set aside.

Cook pasta according to package directions. Drain and rinse under cold water. Add the broccoli, snow peas, corn, olives, and the dressing and toss until well combined. If desired, add tuna fish and/ or feta cheese and stir to combine. The salad can be served immediately or refrigerated for several hours before serving.

*The vegetables may be served raw or lightly blanched. If blanching, bring 6 cups of water to a boil in a sauce pot. Drop vegetables in boiling water for 30 seconds to 1 minute. Drain immediately and rinse under cold water to stop the cooking process.

nutritional wisdom
mindful eating
by Aruni Nan Futuronsky, life coach

Eating mindfully—being present in the chewing and the tasting of your food—
is a powerful way to practice being in the moment and to fully enjoy healthful
foods. Practice mindfully eating one meal a day. Watch your world change.

Mindfulness practice:

- Develops our capacity to be aware
- Teaches us how to inhabit the present moment
- Purposefully directs our attention to what is
- Helps us to release old, automatic responses
- Releases self-judgment
- Cultivates new capacity in us to respond differently to life.

Mindful eating is:

- The practice of being in the moment in body, mind, and spirit while eating
- A state of focused and relaxed awareness
- Grounded in non-judgmental compassion
- An ancient technique of self-nurturance
- An ongoing practice of radical self-acceptance balanced with right action.

Mindful eating helps you:

- Connect with your body's innate wisdom and knowing
- Realign with your body's signals and messages
- Create non-habitual, "sacred" time for yourself
- Strengthen the witness, the capacity to observe and attend to self
- Create effective choices for new behavior.

dressings

A salad without dressing is like a day without sunshine, a rainstorm without an umbrella, or—worse still—a cake without frosting! At Kripalu, we love to give our guests plenty of variety, so we offer six or more dressings each day. Kept in the refrigerator, our homemade dressings with fresh vegetables or fruit (such as our Ume Scallion or Raspberry Walnut dressings) stay fresh for five days, while the others last for up to two weeks. Since olive oil will solidify when cooled, it's a good idea to remove the dressings from the refrigerator about 15 minutes before serving, or give the bottle a really good shake. If extra-virgin olive oil is over processed, it will develop an undesirable bitter flavor, so when making these dressings, only blend until well combined.

kripalu house dressing

Makes about 1 1/2 cups

1/4 cup tahini
2 tablespoons fresh lemon juice
1 tablespoon tamari
1 teaspoon toasted sesame oil
1 teaspoon minced garlic
1/2 teaspoon mustard powder
1/2 teaspoon chili powder
1/4 teaspoon sea salt
Pinch of cayenne pepper
3/4 cup extra-virgin olive oil
1/2 cup water

This dressing can be made in a regular blender or with an immersion blender. Place all the ingredients except the olive oil and 1/4 cup of the water in a blender jar (or a mixing bowl if using an immersion blender). Pulse until well combined. Add the oil and pulse briefly, just until incorporated. Add the remaining water and pulse briefly until the desired consistency is reached.

ume scallion dressing

Makes about 1 1/2 cups

4–5 scallions, chopped
1/2 cup water
1 tablespoon umeboshi plum vinegar
1 cup extra-virgin olive oil

Place scallions, water, and vinegar in blender and process until smooth. Add the oil and pulse briefly, just until incorporated.

feta dressing

Makes about 2 1/2 cups

1/2 cup Veganaise™ (egg-less mayonnaise)
1/2 cup water
2 1/2 tablespoons fresh lemon juice
2 tablespoons minced fresh parsley
1 tablespoon minced garlic
1/4 teaspoon sea salt
1 cup extra-virgin olive oil
1 cup crumbled feta cheese

This dressing can be made in a regular blender or with an immersion blender. Place all the ingredients except the olive oil and 1/4 cup of the feta cheese in a blender jar (or a mixing bowl if using an immersion blender). Pulse until well combined. Add the oil and remaining feta and pulse briefly, just until incorporated.

clockwise from top left:
ume scallion dressing
feta dressing
raspberry walnut dressing
kripalu house dressing
lemon garlic dressing
honey dijon dressing
balsamic vinaigrette

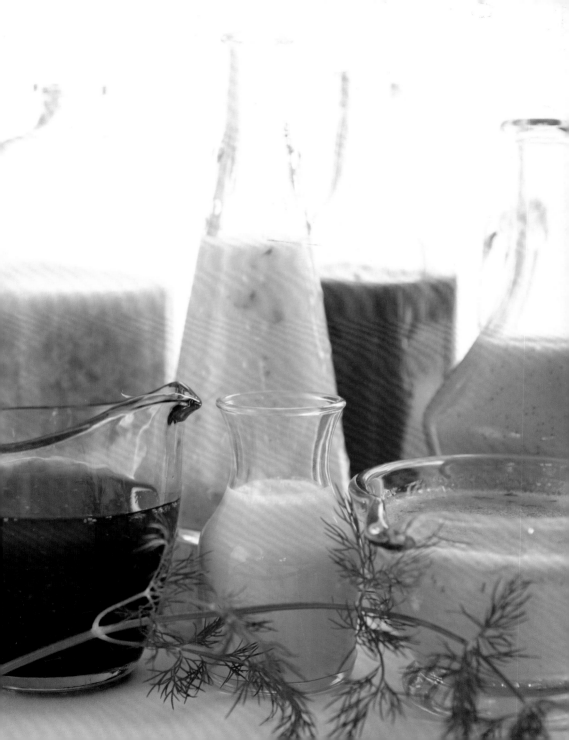

honey dijon dressing

Makes 1 cup

1/4 cup Veganaise™ (egg-less mayonnaise)
1/4 cup Dijon mustard
1/4 cup honey
1/4 cup water

Whisk the ingredients together in a medium mixing bowl.

balsamic vinaigrette

Makes about 1 1/4 cups

1 cup extra-virgin olive oil
1/4 cup balsamic vinegar
1 teaspoon dried oregano
1/4 teaspoon sea salt
Pinch of black pepper

Whisk the ingredients together in a medium mixing bowl or place in a salad dressing container and shake to blend.

lemon garlic dressing

Makes about 2 1/4 cups

1 cup water
3/4 cup fresh lemon juice
1/2 cup extra-virgin olive oil
2 tablespoons minced garlic
1 tablespoon minced fresh dill
1/2 teaspoon sea salt

Whisk the ingredients together in a medium mixing bowl or place in a salad dressing container and shake to blend.

raspberry walnut dressing

Makes about 1 1/2 cups

1/2 cup frozen raspberries, thawed
3 tablespoons white wine vinegar
1 1/2 teaspoons Dijon mustard
2 tablespoons honey
1/2 teaspoon sea salt
Pinch of black pepper
1/4 cup water
1/2 cup extra-virgin olive oil or walnut oil
1/4 cup chopped walnuts

Place all the ingredients except the olive oil and walnuts in a blender jar. Pulse until well combined. Add the oil and walnuts and pulse briefly, just until incorporated.

sandwiches

The sandwich, in its many forms, has always stood out as a classic food. You simply can't go wrong when assembling your favorite creation, whether it contains hot or cold fillings; has fresh, toasted, or grilled bread; or uses lots of add-ins and condiments or just one ingredient. The sandwich is so well loved that even those who want to forego the bread entirely are finding great satisfaction wrapping their favorite fillings in lightly steamed greens or crisp lettuce leaves. So get creative and see what fun combinations and new sandwich concepts you can make using our recipes as a starting point.

hot sandwiches

We've created four healthful takes on the hot sandwich for you to try. Reubens are a classic and we love our vegan version of the sauce even on a nonvegetarian sandwich. The Middle Eastern Lentil or Turkey Kibbee served in pita bread or on top of our quinoa tabouli with one of our sauces makes for a spicy option. Consider the festive fajita sandwich when you're having guests for lunch or dinner, as it's easily tailored to individuals' preferences. And be sure to try our Sloppy Joes. Wow, that's a sandwich!

chicken or tofu fajitas with sautéed vegetables, pineapple salsa, tomatillo salsa, and guacamole

Serves 4

Chicken or Tofu Fajitas (recipe follows)
Sautéed Vegetables (recipe follows)
Pineapple Salsa (recipe follows)
Tomatillo Salsa (recipe follows)
Guacamole (recipe follows)
2 cups shredded lettuce
4 fajita wraps, flour tortillas or corn tortillas

Place each component in a serving dish and allow guests to assemble their own fajitas.

chicken or tofu fajitas

for the rub
1/2 teaspoon ground cumin
1/2 teaspoon coriander
1/4 teaspoon chili powder if using chicken,
    1/2 teaspoon if using tofu
1/4 teaspoon cayenne pepper
1/2 teaspoon sea salt

8 ounces boneless chicken breast or 12 ounces
    firm tofu, cut into strips (about 1-inch wide by
    1/4-inch thick)

2 tablespoons grape seed or other high-heat oil,
    plus more if needed
Lime wedges

Combine the spices for the rub. Sprinkle over the chicken or tofu and gently rub in. Set aside for 30 minutes.

Heat the oil in a skillet over medium-high heat, until shimmering. Add chicken or tofu. Cook chicken until it is no longer pink or tofu until it is lightly browned, adding additional oil if needed. When done, drain on paper towels to absorb any excess oil. Place in a serving dish, squeeze a little lime juice over the top and toss gently. (The chicken or tofu may also be grilled.)

*clockwise from back left
sour cream, guacamole, tomatillo
salsa, pineapple salsa, tofu fajita
with sautéed vegetable*

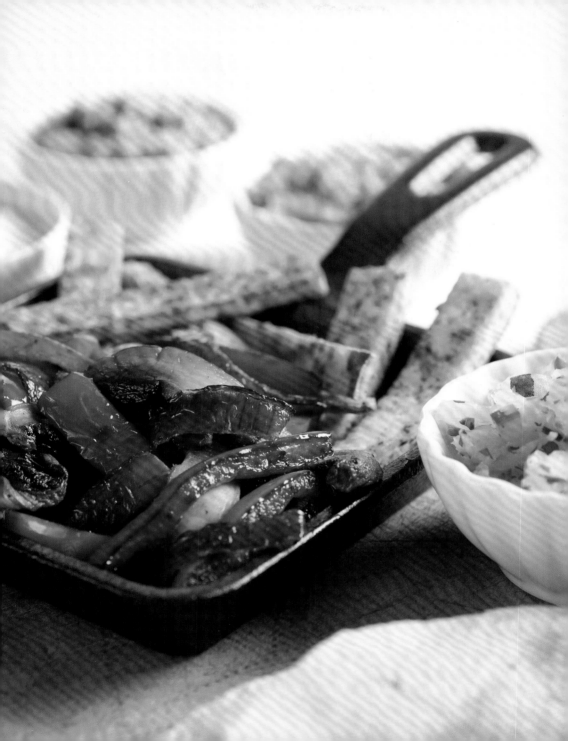

sautéed vegetables

2 teaspoons grape-seed or other high-heat oil
   (more if needed)
1 onion, sliced
1/2 red bell pepper, sliced
1/2 green bell pepper, sliced
4 large mushrooms, sliced
Sea salt as needed

Heat the oil in a skillet over medium-high heat until shimmering. Sauté vegetables separately with a little bit of salt, adding more oil as needed. When done, drain on paper towels to absorb any excess oil. Combine sautéed vegetables in a serving dish.

Note Other vegetables may be used, so get creative! Zucchini and summer squash are particularly nice in fajitas. All vegetables can be grilled instead of sautéed.

tomatillo salsa

Makes 1 cup

2 cups diced fresh tomatillos
1/4 cup diced red onion
2 tablespoons minced fresh cilantro
2 teaspoons fresh lime juice
1 teaspoon minced garlic
1 teaspoon minced jalapeno or more to taste
1/4 teaspoon sea salt, plus more to taste

Place tomatillos in a small saucepan. Cook gently for 10 minutes until soft.

Place cooked tomatillos in the bowl of a food processor with the remaining ingredients. Blend to desired chunkiness. Transfer to a serving bowl. Taste and add more salt if desired.

pineapple salsa

Makes 2 cups

1 1/2 cups crushed pineapple, drained
2 tablespoons diced red onion
1 tablespoon minced fresh cilantro
Pinch of coriander
1/4 cup diced green bell peppers
1 tablespoon minced garlic
1 teaspoon minced jalapeno or more to taste
Pinch of sea salt
Pinch of black pepper

Combine the ingredients in a medium mixing bowl and stir to combine. Set aside for 30 minutes before serving. Serve chilled or at room temperature.

guacamole

Makes about 1 1/2 cups

2 ripe avocados
2 tablespoons extra-virgin olive oil
1/4 cup fresh lemon juice
1/4 cup chopped tomatoes, drained (optional)
2 tablespoons minced red onion
1 tablespoon minced fresh cilantro
1 tablespoon minced garlic
1/4 teaspoon sea salt

In a medium-size bowl, mash avocados with a fork to desired consistency. Add the remaining ingredients and mix until well blended. Transfer to a serving bowl and serve immediately.

reuben sandwiches with tempeh or turkey

Makes 4 sandwiches

reuben sauce
3/4 cup Veganaise™ (egg-less mayonnaise)
1/4 cup ketchup
2 tablespoons capers
1 teaspoon bottled hot sauce
1/2 teaspoon minced garlic
Pinch of sea salt

tempeh for reuben sandwiches
1 8-ounce package tempeh, cut in half lengthwise
    and then widthwise to make 4 pieces
2 cups water
2 tablespoons Bragg Liquid Aminos™
    (all-purpose seasoning) or tamari

turkey for reuben sandwiches
8 ounces sliced all-natural turkey meat (preferably
    nitrate- and preservative-free)

sandwiches
1 recipe Reuben Sauce
Baked tempeh strips or turkey slices
4 slices Swiss cheese
8 slices rye bread
1 cup sauerkraut (preferably naturally fermented)
Butter or Earth Balance™ (vegan spread) for
    grilling

make the reuben sauce
Whisk the ingredients together in a medium mixing bowl and set aside.

prepare the tempeh (if using)
To make tempeh more digestible, it's best to steam it before its final preparation. Place tempeh in a steamer basket and place in a pot with about 1 inch of water. Cover, bring to a boil, and steam for 15 minutes

Combine the water and Bragg Liquid Aminos™ or tamari. Add the steamed tempeh and marinate for at least 30 minutes and up to 3 hours. Drain the tempeh well. Place the tempeh on an oiled baking sheet and blot dry. Bake in a 350-degree oven for 15 minutes, flipping halfway through cooking.

assemble and grill the sandwiches:
Spread 1 tablespoon of Reuben Sauce on each of the 8 slices of bread. Serve remaining sauce on the side or save for future use.

Divide tempeh or turkey slices between 4 slices of bread and top each with one slice of cheese, 1/4 cup sauerkraut, and a slice of bread. Butter and grill the sandwiches until the cheese is melted.

tempeh or turkey sloppy joes

Serves 2–4

Sloppy Joe Sauce (recipe follows)
Cooked tempeh or turkey
2–4 hamburger buns

tempeh version

1 tablespoon extra-virgin olive oil
8 ounces of tempeh, crumbled

turkey version

1 tablespoon extra-virgin olive oil
1/2 pound ground turkey

sloppy joe sauce

2 tablespoons extra-virgin olive oil
1 small onion, diced
1 green bell pepper, diced
2 tablespoons minced garlic
1/4 cup tomato paste
1 14-ounce can tomato puree
2 tablespoons mustard, preferably stone ground
2 tablespoons molasses
2 teaspoons chili powder
1 teaspoon ground cumin
1 teaspoon sea salt
1/8 teaspoon dried thyme
1/8 teaspoon black pepper
Water, as needed

to prepare the tempeh

To make tempeh more digestible, it's best to steam it before its final preparation. Place crumbled tempeh in a steamer basket and place in a pot with about 1-inch of water. Cover, bring to a boil, and steam for 15 minutes.

Heat the oil in a skillet over medium heat until shimmering. Add the tempeh and cook, stirring, until lightly browned. Set aside.

to prepare the turkey

Heat the oil in a skillet over medium heat until shimmering. Add the turkey and cook until no longer pink. Depending on how lean the turkey is, you may need more oil. If it seems too oily, drain before serving. Set aside.

to make the sloppy joe sauce

Heat the oil in a skillet over medium heat until shimmering. Add onions and cook until caramelized. Add peppers and sauté until soft. Add garlic and simmer for 5 minutes more. Add tomato paste and sauté for 2 to 3 minutes until it starts to stick to the bottom of the pan. Deglaze with a little water, white wine, or stock. Add remaining ingredients and mix well. Add cooked turkey or tempeh and gently simmer, stirring occasionally, for 10 minutes. If mixture seems too thick, add a little water.

to finish the sandwiches

Split each hamburger bun and fill with the Sloppy Joe Sauce with tempeh or turkey. Serve hot.

turkey or lentil kibbee in pita with yogurt cucumber sauce and tahini sauce

Serves 4

Lentil or Turkey Kibbee (recipes follow)
4 pita pockets
Tahini Sauce (recipe follows)
Yogurt Cucumber Sauce (recipe follows)
Extra-virgin olive oil, shredded lettuce, chopped
    red onion (optional)

Place 3 balls of Lentil or Turkey Kibbee in a pita pocket. Serve with your choice of yogurt cucumber or tahini sauce. Alternately, you can serve the kibbee with a little olive oil, shredded lettuce, and chopped red onion.

turkey kibbee

1/2 cup pine nuts
1/2 pound ground turkey
1/4 cup minced onion
1 teaspoon cinnamon
1/2 teaspoon allspice
1/2 teaspoon sea salt
Pinch of black pepper
Extra-virgin olive oil, as need for baking

Preheat oven to 350 degrees.

Toast pine nuts in small skillet over medium heat until lightly browned. Stir constantly to avoid burning. Cool. Transfer to a food processor and pulse until finely ground.

Place the ground pine nuts in a large mixing bowl with the remaining ingredients, except the oil. Stir until mixture is well combined. Divide into 12 portions, roll into balls, and place on an oiled baking sheet. Bake until turkey is cooked through and no longer pink, about 20 minutes.

lentil kibbee

1/2 cup pine nuts
1/2 cup green lentils
2 cups water
1 medium boiling potato, peeled and cubed
1/4 cup finely ground flaxseed
1 tablespoon extra-virgin olive oil, plus
    more for baking
1 teaspoon cinnamon
1/2 teaspoon allspice
1/2 teaspoon sea salt
Pinch of black pepper

Toast pine nuts in small skillet over medium heat until lightly browned. Stir constantly to avoid burning. Cool. Transfer to a food processor and pulse until finely ground. Set aside.

Place lentils in a sauce pot with the water. Bring to a boil, then reduce heat, partially cover, and simmer until lentils are soft but still intact, 20 to 30 minutes. Drain well. Spread on platter to cool.

While lentils are cooking, steam potatoes (boiling will make them too wet) until tender, drain, pat dry, and cool.

Preheat oven to 350 degrees.

Put the lentils, potatoes, pine nuts and remaining ingredients in the bowl of a food processor. Pulse just until mixture comes together. Divide into 12 portions, roll into balls, and place on an oiled baking sheet. Spray or brush a little oil on top of the kibbee balls. Bake for 20 minutes.

tahini sauce

Makes about 3/4 cup

1/3 cup plus 1 tablespoon water
1/3 cup tahini
3 tablespoons fresh lemon juice
1/2 teaspoon minced garlic
Pinch of sea salt
Pinch of ground cumin

Place all ingredients in a blender and process until smooth. Adjust seasonings to taste.

Note Sauce will thicken overnight; just add more water to thin it out.

yogurt cucumber sauce

Makes about 1 1/4 cups

3/4 cup plain yogurt
1/2 cup grated cucumber
2 tablespoons fresh lemon juice
1 tablespoon minced fresh mint
1/4 teaspoon ground cumin
Pinch of ground coriander
Pinch of sea salt
Pinch of black pepper

Whisk all ingredients together in a medium mixing bowl. Chill before serving.

Note For a thicker yogurt sauce, drain the yogurt through a cheesecloth for 20 minutes, or try using a Greek-style yogurt instead.

paninis—fabulous grilled sandwich combinations

Here are some great combinations to try out in your panini press or stovetop griddle. Fill whole-grain bread slices, split ciabatta rolls, or wraps with any of the following combinations—including some recipes found throughout this book!

- Tomato, fresh mozzarella, and basil with a splash of extra-virgin olive oil

- Hummus (see recipe on page 40), arugula, and roasted red peppers

- Grilled summer vegetables, goat cheese, and Tapenade (see recipe on page 44)

- Vegan Hazelnut Cocoa Spread or Almond Cocoa Spread (see recipes on page 44) with banana and cinnamon

- Tuna, spinach, and cheddar cheese (pictured at right)

- Grilled chicken or tofu, pesto, and arugula

- Mexican Black Bean Salad (see recipe on page 20), jack cheese, salsa

- Hummus, Quinoa Tabouli Salad (see recipe on page 19), and red bell peppers

panini with tuna apple walnut salad, spinach, and cheddar cheese

34

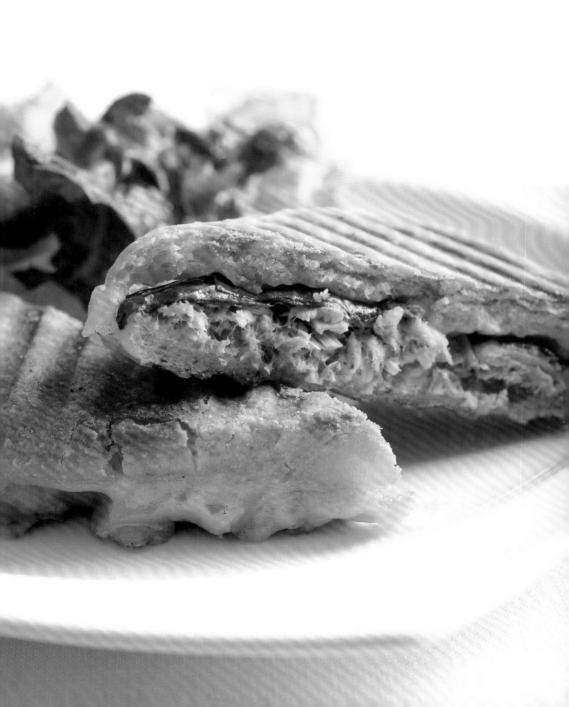

cold sandwiches

Several years ago, Kripalu opened a create-your-own sandwich bar buffet (complete with panini grill) as a meal alternative for lunch and dinner. The bar's endless versatility made it an instant crowd pleaser. Here are some of our favorite recipes, along with some of our favorite panini offerings. Remember to use organic or natural chicken and eggs and dolphin-safe, unsalted tuna for a more healthful sandwich—and healthier planet. We love to use the mayonnaise substitute Vegenaise™, and it's available in most natural foods stores in the refrigerated section. If it's not available in your area, simply use the best-quality, all-natural mayonnaise or substitute you can find.

chicken salad sandwiches three ways

**Mint, Grape, and Cashew Chicken Salad;
Curry Chicken Salad;
Tarragon Chicken Salad**

Serves 2

1/2 pound boneless chicken meat, cooked, cut
    into 1-inch pieces, cooled
or 2 cups leftover cooked, diced chicken meat
Your choice: Mint, Grape, and Cashew Dressing,
    Curry Dressing, Tarragon-Sour Cream
    Dressing, or (recipes follow)
4 slices whole grain bread
Lettuce, tomato, sprouts (optional)

dressing for mint, grape, cashew chicken salad
1/4 cup sliced grapes
3 tablespoons extra-virgin olive oil
3 tablespoons roasted cashew pieces
2 tablespoons minced fresh mint
2 tablespoons fresh lemon juice
1 tablespoon Dijon mustard
1 tablespoon honey
1/4 teaspoon sea salt
Pinch of black pepper

Whisk ingredients together in a large mixing bowl.

dressing for curry chicken salad
1/2 cup Vegenaise™ (egg-less mayonnaise)
1 stalk celery, diced fine
2 teaspoons agave nectar
1/2 teaspoon curry powder
1/2 teaspoon garlic powder
1/2 teaspoon sea salt
Pinch of black pepper

Whisk ingredients together in a large mixing bowl

dressing for tarragon chicken salad
1/2 cup Vegenaise™ (egg-less mayonnaise)
2 stalks celery, diced fine
3 tablespoons sour cream
1 tablespoon minced fresh tarragon
1 tablespoon tarragon vinegar
1/2 teaspoon dried tarragon
1/2 teaspoon sea salt

Whisk ingredients together in a large mixing bowl

assemble chicken salad
Add cooled, cubed chicken to your choice of
dressing and mix until thoroughly combined. Chill
before serving.

assemble sandwiches
Divide the chicken salad between two slices of
bread. Top with lettuce, tomato, and sprouts if using.
Top with two slices of bread and serve immediately.

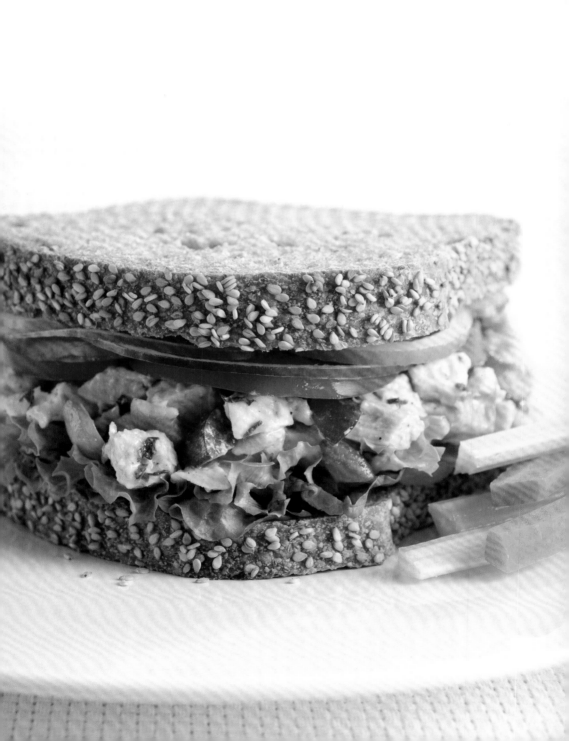

tuna apple walnut salad

Serves 2

1 6-ounce can of unsalted, water-packed tuna,
   drained
1 stalk celery, diced
1/2 small apple, diced
1/4 cup chopped walnuts
1/4 cup Veganaise™ (egg-less mayonnaise)
2 tablespoons minced fresh parsley
Pinch of black pepper
Pinch of sea salt

Combine all ingredients in a mixing bowl and stir
until thoroughly combined. Chill before serving.

chickpea of the sea

Serves 4

1 13-ounce can of garbanzo beans (chickpeas),
   drained or 1 1/4 cups cooked garbanzo beans
1 stalk celery, finely chopped
2 scallions, finely sliced
2 tablespoons extra-virgin olive oil
1 1/2 teaspoons apple cider vinegar
1 teaspoon umeboshi plum vinegar
1 tablespoon nutritional yeast
1/4 teaspoon celery seed
Pinch of sea salt, or to taste
Pinch of cayenne pepper
Pinch of black pepper

Combine all ingredients in food processor. Pulse
until about half of the chickpeas are mashed, or
until desired consistency is reached, scraping
down sides of the bowl as necessary. Chill before
serving.

curry tofu salad

Serves 4

for the dressing
1/2 cup Veganaise™ (egg-less mayonnaise)
2 teaspoons mustard, preferably stone ground
1 1/2 teaspoons curry powder
1/2 teaspoon sea salt

for the salad
1 pound firm tofu, crumbled
1 stalk celery, diced fine
1/4 cup roasted sunflower seeds
1/4 cup grated carrots
2 scallions, sliced

Sliced red bell pepper (optional)
Sprouts (optional)

Whisk the dressing ingredients together in a large
mixing bowl. Add the salad ingredients and mix
until thoroughly blended. Chill before serving.
Use the Curry Tofu Salad in a sandwich with your
favorite bread or roll up with red bell pepper slice
and sprouts in lettuce leaves to make "wraps."
(See photo).

curry tofu sala

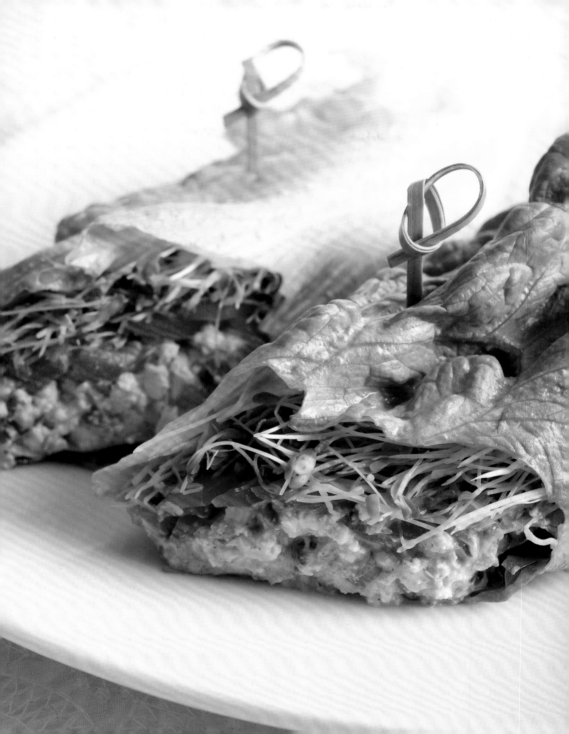

baba ghanoush

Makes about 1 1/2 cups

1 large eggplant
1/3 cup tahini
3 tablespoons fresh lemon juice
1 1/2 tablespoons minced garlic
1 tablespoon extra-virgin olive oil
1/2 teaspoon sea salt

for serving

Sliced bread if using for sandwiches or toasted
    pita chips and sliced vegetables if serving as
    a dip
Minced fresh parsley for garnish (optional)
Extra-virgin olive oil

Preheat oven to 375 degrees. Cut eggplant in half
and place on a baking sheet and roast until soft,
20 to 30 minutes. When eggplant is cool enough
to handle, remove the skin and discard. Measure
out 1 cup of cooked eggplant (reserving any extra
for another use) and place in the bowl of a food
processor. Add remaining ingredients and blend
until creamy, scraping down sides of the bowl as
necessary. Chill for at least 3 hours.

Use the Baba Ghanoush to make sandwiches
or as a dip with toasted pita chips and sliced
vegetables. Transfer to a serving bowl and drizzle
with a little olive oil and garnish with the minced
parsley if desired.

hummus

Makes about 2 cups

1 15-ounce can of garbanzo beans (chickpeas),
    drained or 1 1/4 cups cooked garbanzo beans
1/4 cup tahini
1/4 cup fresh lemon juice
3 to 4 tablespoons water
2 tablespoons extra-virgin olive oil
1 tablespoon minced garlic
1/2 teaspoon sea salt
Pinch of ground cumin
Pinch of ground coriander

for serving

Sliced bread if using for sandwiches or toasted pita
    chips and sliced vegetables if serving as a dip
Minced fresh parsley for garnish (optional)
Extra-virgin olive oil

Place all the hummus ingredients in the bowl of a
food processor. Blend until creamy, scraping down
sides of the bowl as necessary. Use the hummus
to make sandwiches or as a dip with toasted pita
chips and sliced vegetables. Transfer to a serving
bowl and drizzle with a little olive oil and garnish
with the minced parsley if desired.

egg salad

Serves 4

6 hard-boiled eggs, peeled
1/3 cup Veganaise™ (egg-less mayonnaise)
2 scallions, sliced
2 tablespoons minced fresh parsley
2 tablespoons dill relish (or minced dill pickle)
1/2 teaspoon mustard powder (optional)
1/4 teaspoon sea salt
Pinch of black pepper

Finely dice the hard-boiled eggs. Place in a large
mixing bowl with the remaining ingredients and
mix until thoroughly combined. Chill before serving.

nutritional wisdom
grow what you can
John Bagnulo, MPH, PhD, nutrition and fitness instructor

Personal gardens yield more than a bounty of crops; they provide stress reduction, an opportunity for moderate exercise, and a place to meditate and reconnect with nature. In terms of nutrition, there's little doubt that personal gardens offer enormous health benefits, since we increase our consumption of fruits and vegetables when it's easy to stroll outside and harvest them.

Research shows that the nutrient density of commercially grown fruits and vegetables has been in steady decline. Bred for maximum yield and the ability to withstand transportation and long stays in grocery stores, most fruits and vegetables have lost a major percentage of their vitamins and minerals. Most of us have tasted an exceptional tomato fresh from a friend's garden. The same sublime taste can be experienced with innumerable, non-commercially grown fruits and vegetables, such as spinach, strawberries, and carrots.

When we choose to plant a small garden or have a few pots to grow vegetable or berry plants, we get the added benefit of controlling the quality of that soil. Something as simple as the addition of compost to your garden soil can give it a major boost, and the nutritional payoff can be great.

If you'd like to start a small garden, opt for low-maintenance greens that are high in beneficial nutrients, such as Swiss chard or rainbow chard. I also recommend giving butternut squash a try. The Waltham variety is so sweet that with a little cinnamon it could pass as dessert. Whatever you choose to grow will nourish you in a number of ways, so let your creative juices flow.

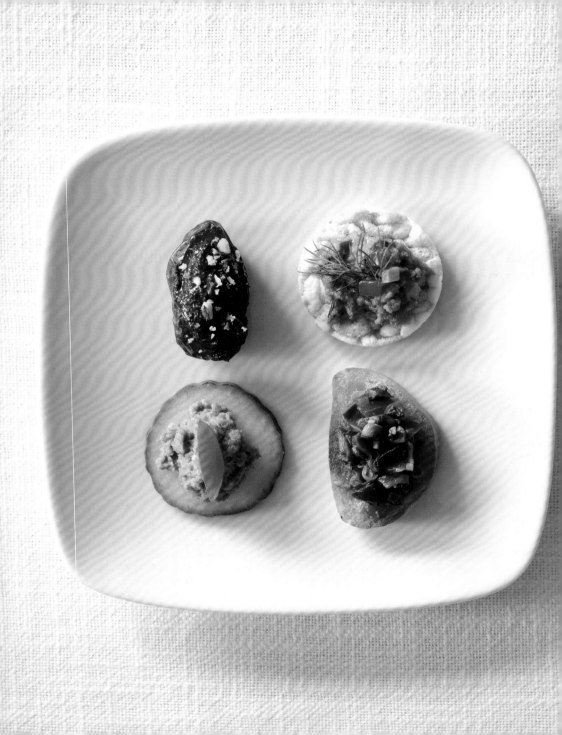

spreads (savory and sweet)

Whether savory or sweet, spreads offer great versatility and flavor. Each of these spreads does just fine standing on its own as a topper to rice cakes, toast, or vegetables. But we invite you to get creative and make some fun sandwich combinations pairing them with grilled chicken or tofu, or raw or grilled vegetables. Or how about a banana and Vegan Hazelnut Cocoa Spread panini?

cinnamon raisin tahini miso spread

Makes about 1 1/2 cups

1/4 cup tahini
1/2 cup chopped raisins
1/4 cup water
3 tablespoons agave nectar
2 teaspoons white miso
1/2 teaspoon cinnamon
Pinch of ground ginger
2 tablespoons finely chopped walnuts

for serving
Whole grain sliced bread, sliced baguette,
    or rice cakes

Place all ingredients except the walnuts in a blender. Blend until creamy, scraping down sides of the blender as necessary. Transfer mixture to a medium mixing bowl and fold in the walnuts.

Serve the spread on whole-grain sliced bread, sliced baguette, or rice cakes.

savory tahini miso spread

Makes about 1 1/2 cups

1/2 cup tahini
2 teaspoons white miso
3 tablespoons minced red onion
2 tablespoons minced red bell pepper
2 tablespoons minced carrot
2 tablespoons soaked and minced sun-dried
    tomatoes
3 tablespoons water
1 teaspoon agave nectar
1 1/2 tablespoons minced fresh chives
1 tablespoon minced fresh dill
Pinch of garlic powder

for serving
Crostini, rice crackers, rice cakes, toasted pita
    chips, or cucumber slices

Place tahini, miso, and 1 tablespoon each of the red onion, red pepper, and carrot in the bowl of a food processor. Add the sun-dried tomatoes, water, and agave and blend until smooth, scraping down sides of the bowl as necessary. Transfer mixture into medium mixing bowl. Fold in the chives, dill, garlic powder, and remaining red onion, red pepper, and carrot.

Serve the spread on crostini, rice crackers, rice cakes, toasted pita chips, or cucumber slices.

*Clockwise from top left:
vegan hazelnut cocoa spread,
savory tahini miso spread, tapenade,
carrot sunflower spread*

tapenade

Makes 1 cup

1 cup pitted kalamata olives, drained
1 1/2 tablespoons fresh lemon juice
1 tablespoon minced garlic
1 tablespoon capers, drained
1 tablespoon extra-virgin olive oil
1/2 roasted red bell pepper, finely diced (optional)

for serving

Crostini, rice crackers, rice cakes, toasted pita
  chips, or cucumber slices

Place all the tapenade ingredients in food processor and pulse until desired consistency is reached.
(See photo on page 42.)

Serve the spread on crostini, rice crackers, rice
cakes, toasted pita chips, or cucumber slices.

vegan hazelnut cocoa spread

Makes about 1 1/4 cups

1/2 cup ground raw hazelnut meal (grind whole
  hazelnuts in food processor until finely ground,
  then measure)
1/4 cup plus 1 tablespoon cocoa powder
1/4 cup plus 1 tablespoon agave nectar
3 tablespoons soy milk
Pinch of sea salt

for serving

Rice cakes or whole-grain sliced bread
Sliced banana (optional)

Place ingredients in a food processor. Blend until
creamy, scraping down sides of the bowl if necessary.

Serve the spread on rice cakes or bread, plain or
toasted. Top with banana slices if desired.

carrot sunflower spread

Makes about 1 1/2 cups

2 cups medium-diced carrots
1 cup toasted sunflower seeds
2 tablespoons nutritional yeast
2 tablespoons tamari

for serving

Crostini, rice crackers, rice cakes, toasted pita
  chips, or cucumber slices

Boil carrots until tender. Drain and cool.

Place sunflower seeds in the bowl of a food
processor. Process just until finely ground. Add
the cooked carrots, yeast, and tamari and process
until desired consistency is reached, occasionally
scraping down the sides of the bowl as necessary.

Serve the spread on crostini, rice crackers, rice
cakes, toasted pita chips, or cucumber slices.

almond cocoa spread

Makes about 1 cup

1/2 cup creamy almond butter
1/4 cup plus 1 tablespoon cocoa powder
1/4 cup plus 1 tablespoon agave nectar
1 tablespoon plain dairy or soy yogurt

for serving

Rice cakes or whole-grain sliced bread

Place ingredients in a food processor. Blend
until creamy, scraping down sides of the bowl if
necessary.

Serve the spread on rice cakes or bread, plain or
toasted.

soups

Soups don't have to disappear from your menu just because it's summer. Soups are one of the Kripalu menu items that receive the most compliments year-round. The key is to keep them light, not overcooked (if cooked at all) and uplifting in flavor. Fresh herbs are the best way to accomplish this and we use an abundance of them in all our dishes.

cold soups

Most of these soups never actually get cooked at all. This makes them not only cooling and refreshing, but also quick and easy. Cold soups refrigerate nicely and can be enjoyed any time of day. The Raw Avocado Soup, however, is one recipe that needs to be eaten immediately, as leftovers don't hold up well. If the weather turns cool, the Borscht is just as nice served hot with a dollop of sour cream on top.

raw avocado soup

Serves 4

2 1/2 cups water, plus more as needed
2 cups chopped romaine lettuce
2 cups diced cucumber
2 ripe avocados, pitted and flesh scooped out
2 scallions, roughly chopped
3 tablespoons fresh lemon juice
3 tablespoons minced fresh mint, plus more for
  garnish
1 tablespoon extra-virgin olive oil
1 tablespoon minced garlic
1 teaspoon sea salt

Place all the ingredients in blender and puree until smooth, adding more water if needed. Serve immediately, garnished with mint if desired.

mango yogurt soup

Serves 2–4

2 1/2 cups diced fresh mango
  (or frozen mango, thawed)
2 cups plain yogurt
1/2 cup whole milk
3 tablespoons fresh lime juice
2 tablespoons minced fresh mint,
  plus more for garnish
2 tablespoons minced fresh cilantro,
  plus more for garnish
1 tablespoon agave nectar
1 tablespoon minced ginger
1/4 teaspoon sea salt
Pinch of allspice

Place all ingredients in blender and puree until smooth. Refrigerate until cold. Serve chilled, garnished with mint or cilantro if desired.

clockwise from top le
borscht, mango yogurt sou
raw avocado sou

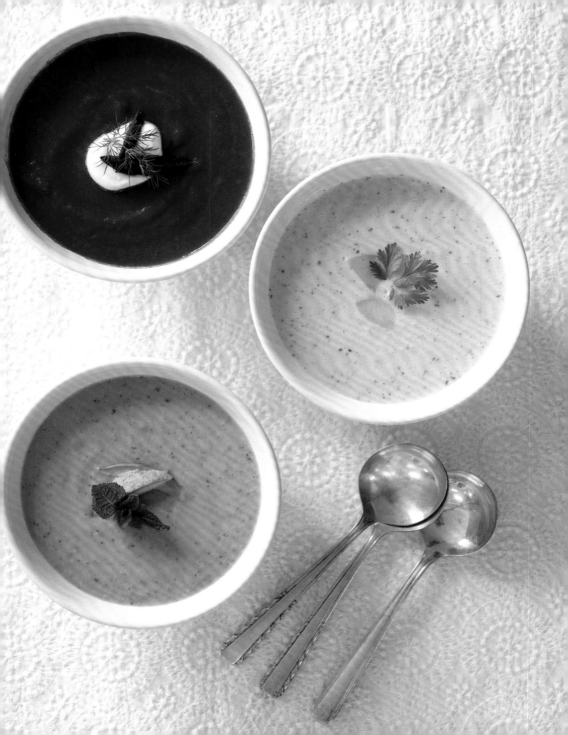

gazpacho

Serves 2–4

3 cups diced tomatoes
1 cup finely diced cucumber
3/4 cup water or vegetable stock,
     plus more as needed
1/2 cup diced red bell pepper
1/2 cup diced green bell pepper
1/4 cup finely diced red onion
2 scallions, diced
2 tablespoons extra-virgin olive oil
1 tablespoon red wine vinegar
1 1/2 teaspoons minced garlic
1/2 teaspoon bottled hot sauce
1/2 teaspoon Worcestershire sauce
1/2 teaspoon sea salt
Pinch of black pepper

Place all ingredients in a blender and puree to de-sired consistency, adding water if needed. Serve chilled or at room temperature.

thai three melon soup

Serves 2–4

1 cup diced seedless watermelon
1 cup diced cantaloupe
1 cup diced honeydew
1 tablespoon minced ginger
1 tablespoon fresh lime juice
Pinch of sea salt

Place ingredients in a soup pot or large bowl and use an immersion blender to process until smooth. Alternatively, place all ingredients in blender and puree until smooth. Serve chilled.

borscht

Serves 4

2 tablespoons extra-virgin olive oil
1/4 cup diced onion
1 tablespoon minced garlic
3 cups diced beets
1/2 cup diced carrot
1 cup shredded green cabbage
1 teaspoon fennel seed
Pinch of ground star anise
4 cups water or vegetable stock
2 tablespoons minced fresh dill
1 tablespoon minced fresh parsley
2 teaspoons apple cider vinegar
Pinch of black pepper
1/2 teaspoon sea salt
Sour cream (optional)

Heat the oil in a 4-quart soup pot over medium heat until shimmering. Add the onion and sauté until translucent. Add garlic and cook for 1 minute. Add the beets, carrots, cabbage, fennel seed, and star anise and cook, stirring often, for 10 minutes. Add water or stock and simmer gently for 30 minutes.

Use an immersion blender to puree the soup right in the pot or transfer the mixture to a blender and puree until smooth. (Use caution while pureeing hot liquid.) Return the purée to the pan and stir in the dill, parsley, vinegar, salt, and pepper.

Let the soup cool for a while, then refrigerate until cold. Serve chilled, garnished with a dollop of sour cream. (The Borscht can be served hot if desired.)

hot soups

Don't worry—although these soups are hot, they're still refreshing and light and make a wonderful addition to a summer meal. If you prefer them even lighter, simply add more stock and then add more seasonings proportionally. As with other recipes in this book, the key is freshness. While dried herbs and bottled citrus have their places, summer cooking is all about freshness.

tomato basil soup

Serves 4

2 tablespoons extra-virgin olive oil
1 small onion, diced
2 tablespoons minced garlic
2 tablespoons tomato paste
2 tablespoons white wine
4 cups fresh, medium-diced tomatoes
1 14-ounce can tomato puree
1/4 cup minced fresh basil, plus more for garnish
1 tablespoon minced fresh thyme
1/2–1 teaspoon sea salt
Pinch of black pepper
Squeeze of lemon juice

Heat oil in a 4-quart soup pot over medium heat until shimmering. Add onions and sauté until translucent, about 10 minutes. Add garlic and cook for 1 minute. Whisk in the tomato paste and cook until it loses its bright red color and begins to stick to the bottom of the pan. Whisk in wine to deglaze the pan and loosen bits stuck to the bottom of the pan. Stir in the diced tomato and tomato puree and cook until heated through. Add the basil, thyme, salt, pepper, and a squeeze of lemon juice. Cook for a few minutes more and adjust seasoning to taste. Serve hot, garnished with fresh basil if desired.

asparagus soup

Serves 4

1/4 cup raw cashews
4 cups water or vegetable stock
4 cups asparagus pieces (about 1-inch each)
1/2 cup medium diced onion
2 tablespoons extra-virgin olive oil
2 tablespoons minced garlic
1 teaspoon sea salt
1 tablespoon lemon juice

Preheat oven to 425 degrees.

Combine the cashews with the water or stock in a 4 quart soup pot. Bring to a boil, then turn off the heat. Let sit while you prepare the asparagus.

Toss the asparagus, onions, olive oil, garlic, and 1/4 teaspoon salt together in a large mixing bowl. Transfer to a baking sheet and roast in the oven, stirring occasionally, until the asparagus is tender but not too soft, 10 to 12 minutes.

Transfer the boiled cashews and water or stock to a blender. Add 3/4 of the roasted asparagus-onion mixture. Puree until very smooth. Return the mixture to the pot, and add the lemon juice and 3/4 teaspoon salt. Heat gently to desired temperature. Serve hot, garnished with the remaining roasted asparagus-onion mixture.

split pea and herb soup

Serves 4

1 cup split green peas, rinsed and checked
    for stones
6 cups water or vegetable stock
1 tablespoon extra-virgin olive oil
1/4 cup sliced onion
1/2 cup sliced leeks, white and light green part
    only, well-rinsed
2 tablespoons minced garlic
2 cups frozen green peas, thawed
1 tablespoon minced fresh thyme
1 tablespoon minced fresh tarragon
1 tablespoon minced fresh dill
Pinch of black pepper
1/2 teaspoon sea salt

Rinse the split peas in cold water..

Place the split peas in a 4-quart soup pot with the water. Bring to a boil, then reduce heat, partially cover, and simmer until split peas are soft, 20 to 30 minutes (about 45 minutes if not soaked*).

While the split peas are cooking, heat the oil in a skillet over medium heat until shimmering. Add the onions and leeks and sauté until translucent, about 10 minutes. Add garlic and cook for 1 minute. Transfer the onion mixture to the cooked split peas. Stir in 1 1/2 cup of the thawed peas and the thyme, tarragon, dill, and pepper. Cook for 5 minutes stirring often. Taste soup before adding salt. If you've used stock, you may not need additional salt. Add the salt if desired.

Use an immersion blender to puree the soup right in the pot or transfer the mixture to a blender and puree until very smooth. (Use caution while pureeing hot liquid.) Return the pureed soup to the pot, add remaining 1/2 cup of thawed peas, and cook until peas and puree are heated through, about 5 minutes. Serve hot.

*Split peas do not require soaking. However, cooking time will be reduced if peas are soaked for more than 4 hours prior to use.

coconut yam soup

Serves 4

1 tablespoon extra-virgin olive oil
1 cup sliced onion
1 tablespoon minced garlic
1 1/2 tablespoons minced ginger
2 cups diced yams or sweet potatoes
3 cups water or vegetable stock
1 13.5-ounce can coconut milk
1/4 cup diced red bell pepper
1 tablespoon mirin or white wine
1 tablespoon fresh lime juice
1 teaspoon sea salt
1 tablespoon minced fresh cilantro (optional)
Lime wedges (optional)

Heat the oil in a soup pot over medium heat until shimmering. Add the onions and sauté until translucent, about 10 minutes. Add the garlic and ginger and cook for 1 minute. Add the yams and water or stock. Bring to a boil, reduce heat, and simmer until the yams are soft. Remove from the heat.

Stir in the coconut milk, red bell pepper, mirin or white wine, and lime juice. Taste the soup before adding salt. If you've used stock, you may not need additional salt.

Use an immersion blender to puree the soup right in the pot or transfer the mixture to a blender and puree until very smooth. (Use caution while pureeing hot liquid.) Return the pureed soup to the pot, reheating soup if necessary. Serve hot. Pour into individual bowls and garnish with cilantro and a wedge of lime.

summer vegetable garden so

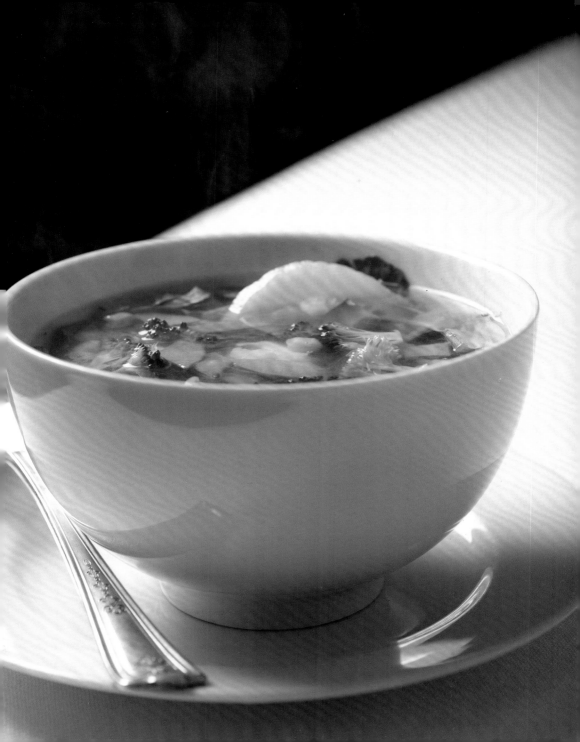

summer garden vegetable soup

Serves 4

6 cups water or vegetable stock
1 carrot, sliced
1/2 cup frozen corn, thawed
1 cup bite-size cauliflower florets
1 cup bite-size broccoli florets
1 cup diagonally cut snow peas
1 cup watercress
1 tablespoon sliced scallions
2 tablespoons minced fresh dill
4 lemon slices
3–4 tablespoons sweet white miso

Bring the water or stock to a boil in a 4 quart soup pot. Add the carrots and simmer until tender, about 5 minutes. Add the corn, cauliflower, and broccoli and cook 1 to 2 minutes until crisp-tender. Add snow peas and cook 1 minute more. Stir in the watercress, scallions, and dill. Turn off heat.

Ladle out one cup of liquid from the soup and put in a small bowl. Whisk in 2 tablespoon of miso until dissolved then stir back into the soup. Taste the soup to determine if it needs more miso. If you've used stock, you may not need additional miso. If you would like more miso, repeat dissolving process with 1 to 2 teaspoons of miso at a time.

Gently reheat soup if needed, being careful not to bring to boil (boiling destroys the beneficial probiotics in miso). Serve hot with a lemon slice in each bowl.

chicken lemongrass soup

Serves 4

8 cups water
1/2 small chicken (half of a chicken will be about 1 1/2 pounds) or
1 1/2 pounds bone-in chicken pieces (preferably white and dark meat)
1 stalk lemongrass, pounded lightly and cut into 2-inch pieces
1 3-inch piece kombu
1 2-inch piece ginger, sliced
2 carrots, sliced
1 small onion, sliced
3 large mushrooms, sliced
1/2 cup bite-size broccoli florets
2 tablespoons tamari
2 scallions, sliced
2 tablespoons minced fresh cilantro
1 tablespoon fresh lime juice
1 teaspoon minced jalapeño

Place water, chicken, lemongrass, kombu, and ginger in a large stock pot. Bring to a boil, reduce heat, and simmer until chicken is cooked through and no longer pink, about 30 minutes. (Skim foam off surface as needed while cooking.) Remove the chicken from stock and set aside to cool.

Strain the stock, discarding solids. Transfer the chicken stock to a 4-quart soup pot and, if necessary, use a ladle to skim off any fat off the surface. Place the pot over medium heat and add the carrots and onions. Simmer until the carrots are tender, about 10 minutes.

When chicken is cool enough to handle, remove the skin. Pull off the meat into bite-size chunks and set aside. Discard the skin and bones.

Add the chicken and mushrooms and simmer for 3 minutes. Add the broccoli and simmer for 1 to 2 minutes more until broccoli is just about at the tenderness you like. Add the tamari, scallions, cilantro, lime juice, and jalapeño and cook 1 minute longer. Adjust seasonings to taste and serve hot.

summer specialty drinks

I believe that tea and herbal drinks are a key part of a healthful diet. Unfortunately, high-sugar, chemical-laden soda has become a staple for many people. Interestingly, sodas do little to actually relieve thirst, and some say they actually increase it. I adore iced tea and herbal drinks in the summertime, and homemade versions are wonderfully inexpensive and tasty alternatives to sodas or bottled teas. Feel free to change, reduce, or remove the recommended sweetener to suit your own taste. And remember to make plenty, as they stay fresh in the refrigerator for days—not that they will last that long!

green tea with lemongrass

Makes 8 cups

8 cups water
6 tea bags of green tea
1 stalk lemongrass, cut into a 6-inch piece and
    pounded slightly
Your choice of sweetener (optional)

Bring the water to a boil in a 4-quart pot. Add
the lemongrass and reduce heat to medium-low.
Simmer for 5 minutes. Remove from heat and add
the tea bags. Steep for 3 to 4 minutes. Strain into
a pitcher and serve as is or sweeten to taste with
your choice of sweetener. Serve hot or chilled.

iced chai

Makes 8 cups

4 tea bags of black tea
3 tablespoons cardamom pods
3 cinnamon sticks
2 tablespoons cloves
2 tablespoons minced ginger
1 tablespoon whole star anise
1 teaspoon whole black peppercorns
4 cups water
4 cups whole milk or soy milk
1/4–1/2 cup sweetener of choice

Place all spices in 4-quart sauce pot and bring
to a boil. Reduce heat and simmer for 5 minutes.
Bring back to a boil, add the black tea, and turn
off heat. Allow to steep for 5 minutes. Strain into a
pitcher and add sweetener to taste. Serve chilled
(or try it hot!)

rosemary rooibos with orange

Makes 8 cups

4 cups water
2 stalks fresh rosemary
7 tea bags of rooibos tea
1 orange, cut into thin slices
1/4 cup orange juice (optional)
4 cups ice

Bring water to a boil in a 4-quart sauce pot.
Remove from heat and add the rosemary and tea
bags. Steep for 5 to 7 minutes, then strain into a
pitcher. Add the orange slices, orange juice (if
using), and ice. The ice will melt, bringing the
tea to the proper strength. Refrigerate until cold.
Serve chilled.

lavender black tea with honey

Makes 8 cups

4 cups water
7 tea bags of English Breakfast tea
3 tablespoons dried lavender
2–4 tablespoons honey
4 cups ice

Bring water to a boil in a 4-quart sauce pot.
Remove from heat and add the tea bags and
lavender. Steep for 5 minutes, then strain into a
pitcher. Stir in the honey and ice. The ice will melt,
bringing the tea to the proper strength. Refrigerate until cold. Serve chilled.

rosemary rooibus with orange

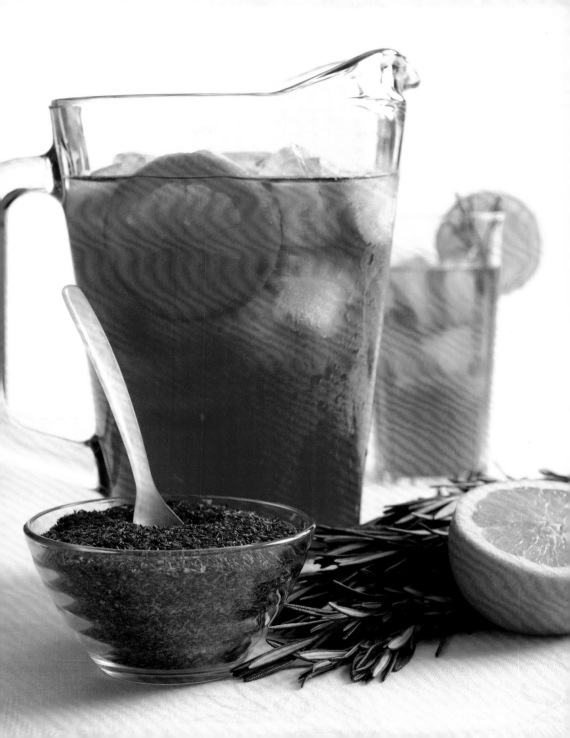

index

Marketing & Communicatons
Tom Rocco, Vice President, Marketing
    and Communications
Elena Erber, Creative Director
Erin Graham Editorial Director
Joyce Monaco, Operations Manager
Derek Hansen, Graphic Designer
Ginger Nicholson, Graphic Designer
Ashley Winseck, Editor
Jonathan Ambar, Editor
Brenda Elling, Marketing Analyst
Lisa Pletzer, Web Content Coordinator
Lyn Meczywor, Marketing Assistant

Special thanks to
Jennifer May, Photographer
Jessica Bard, Food Stylist and
    Recipe Editor
Melissa Jeltsen, Indexer
Qualprint, Pittsfield, Massachusetts

Bon appétit.

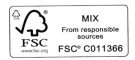